May 2012

PRESIDENT'S EMERGENCY PLAN FOR AIDS RELIEF

Agencies Can Enhance Evaluation Quality, Planning, and Dissemination

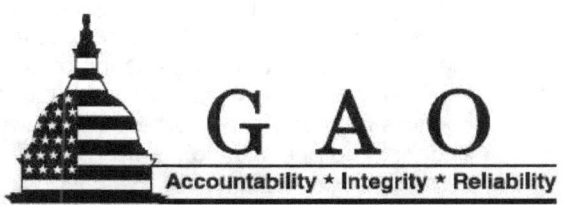

GAO

Accountability ★ Integrity ★ Reliability

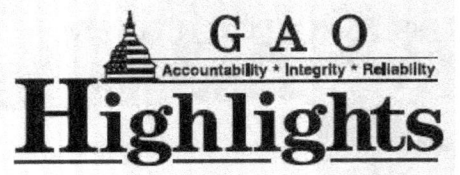

GAO
Accountability * Integrity * Reliability

Highlights

Highlights of GAO-12-673, a report to congressional committees

PRESIDENT'S EMERGENCY PLAN FOR AIDS RELIEF

Agencies Can Enhance Evaluation Quality, Planning, and Dissemination

Why GAO Did This Study

PEPFAR, reauthorized by Congress in fiscal year 2008, supports HIV/AIDS prevention, treatment, and care overseas. The reauthorizing legislation, as well as other U.S. law and government policy, stresses the importance of evaluation for improving program performance, strengthening accountability, and informing decision making. OGAC leads the PEPFAR effort by providing funding and guidance to implementing agencies, primarily CDC and USAID. Responding to legislative mandates, GAO (1) identified PEPFAR evaluation activities and examined the extent to which evaluation findings, conclusions, and recommendations were supported and (2) examined the extent to which PEPFAR policies and procedures adhere to established general evaluation principles. GAO reviewed these principles as well as agencies' policies and guidance; surveyed CDC and USAID officials in 31 PEFAR countries and 3 regions; and analyzed evaluations provided by OGAC, CDC, and USAID.

What GAO Recommends

GAO recommends that State work with CDC and USAID to (1) improve adherence to common evaluation standards, (2) develop PEPFAR evaluation plans, (3) provide guidance for assessing and documenting evaluators' independence and qualifications, and (4) increase online accessibility of evaluation results.

Commenting jointly with HHS's CDC and USAID, State agreed with these recommendations and noted steps it will take to implement them.

View GAO-12-673. For more information, contact David Gootnick at (202) 512-3149 or gootnickd@gao.gov.

What GAO Found

The Department of State's (State) Office of the U.S. Global AIDS Coordinator (OGAC), the Department of Health and Human Services' (HHS) Centers for Disease Control and Prevention (CDC), and the U.S. Agency for International Development (USAID) have evaluated a wide variety of President's Emergency Plan for AIDS Relief (PEPFAR) program activities, demonstrating a clear commitment to evaluation. However, GAO found that the findings, conclusions, and recommendations were not fully supported in many PEPFAR evaluations. Agency officials provided nearly 500 evaluations addressing activities ongoing in fiscal years 2008 through 2010 in all program areas relating to HIV/AIDS treatment, prevention, and care. GAO's assessment of a selected sample of seven OGAC-managed evaluations found that they generally adhered to common evaluation standards, as did most of a selected sample of 15 evaluations managed by CDC and USAID headquarters. Based on this assessment, GAO determined that these evaluations generally contained fully supported findings, conclusions, and recommendations. However, based on a similar assessment of a randomly selected sample taken from 436 evaluations provided by PEPFAR country and regional teams, GAO estimated that 41 percent contained fully supported findings, conclusions, and recommendations, while 44 percent contained partial support and 15 percent were not supported.

Extent to Which Findings, Conclusions, and Recommendations Were Supported in Selected Evaluations

Source of PEPFAR evaluation (number assessed)	Fully supported	Partially supported	Not supported
OGAC-managed evaluations (7 total)	7	0	0
CDC and USAID headquarters evaluations (15 total)	9	6	0
Country and regional team evaluations (436 total)[a]	179 (41 percent)	190 (44 percent)	67 (15 percent)

Source: GAO analysis.

[a]Numbers and percentages reported in this row are estimates based on analysis of 78 evaluations randomly selected from the 436 total. The margin of error associated with proportion estimates is no more than plus or minus 11 percentage points at the 95 percent level of confidence. The margin of error for totals is not more than 44 evaluations.

State, OGAC, CDC, and USAID have established detailed evaluation policies, as recommended by the American Evaluation Association (AEA). However, PEPFAR does not fully adhere to AEA principles relating to evaluation planning, independence and qualifications of evaluators, and public dissemination of evaluation results. Specifically, OGAC does not require country and regional teams to include evaluation plans in their annual operational plans, limiting its ability to ensure that evaluation resources are appropriately targeted. Further, although OGAC, CDC, and USAID evaluation policies and procedures provide some guidance on how to ensure evaluator independence and qualifications, they do not require documentation of these issues. GAO found that most PEPFAR program evaluations did not fully address whether evaluators had conflicts of interest and some did not include detailed information on the identity and makeup of evaluation teams. Finally, although OGAC, CDC, and USAID use a variety of means to share evaluation findings, not all evaluation reports are available online, limiting their accessibility to the public and their usefulness for PEPFAR decision makers, program managers, and other stakeholders.

_____ United States Government Accountability Office

Contents

Figures

Abbreviations

2008 Leadership Act	Tom Lantos and Henry J. Hyde United States Global Leadership Against HIV/AIDS, Tuberculosis, and Malaria Reauthorization Act of 2008
AEA	American Evaluation Association
ARV	antiretroviral
DEC	Development Experience Clearinghouse
DGHA	Division of Global HIV/AIDS
HHS	Department of Health and Human Services
OHA	Office of HIV/AIDS
OGAC	Office of the U.S. Global AIDS Coordinator
PEPFAR	President's Emergency Plan for AIDS Relief
CDC	Centers for Disease Control and Prevention
PHE	public health evaluation
State	Department of State
USAID	U.S. Agency for International Development

This is a work of the U.S. government and is not subject to copyright protection in the United States. The published product may be reproduced and distributed in its entirety without further permission from GAO. However, because this work may contain copyrighted images or other material, permission from the copyright holder may be necessary if you wish to reproduce this material separately.

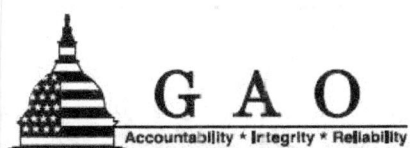

May 31, 2012

Congressional Committees

Through the multibillion-dollar President's Emergency Plan for AIDS Relief (PEPFAR), the United States has supported significant advances in global HIV/AIDS prevention, treatment, and care. Since the program was first authorized in 2003, the estimated number of new HIV infections and AIDS-related deaths has steadily declined while millions of people in low- and middle-income countries have received antiretroviral treatment. Yet for every person placed on treatment, an estimated two people are newly infected with HIV, and the number of people living with HIV expanded from about 28 million in 2001 to 34 million in 2010.

Congress reauthorized PEPFAR in 2008 through passage of the Tom Lantos and Henry J. Hyde United States Global Leadership Against HIV/AIDS, Tuberculosis, and Malaria Reauthorization Act of 2008 (2008 Leadership Act),[1] which sets multiyear targets for prevention, treatment, care, and health systems strengthening programs supported through PEPFAR through fiscal year 2013.[2] The 2008 Leadership Act stated, among other things, that assistance provided to combat HIV/AIDS shall expand impact evaluation and other research and analysis efforts to improve accountability, increase transparency, measure the outcomes and impacts of interventions, ensure the delivery of evidence-based services, and identify and replicate effective models.[3] The Government Performance and Results Act of 1993, amended in 2010 as the Government Performance and Results Modernization Act, also encourages evaluation of federal programs. Moreover, since 2002, the Office of Management and Budget has set expectations for agencies to conduct program evaluations as essential tools for improving program design and operations, determining whether intended outcomes are achieved effectively, and informing decision making.

---

[1]Pub. L. No. 110-293, 122 Stat. 2918.

[2]See Pub. L. No. 110-293, § 101(a).

[3]See Pub. L. No. 110-293, § 301(c)(3).

Responding to requirements in the Consolidated Appropriations Act of 2008 and the 2008 Leadership Act to review global HIV/AIDS program monitoring,[4] this report (1) identifies PEPFAR evaluation activities and examines the extent to which evaluation findings, conclusions, and recommendations are supported and (2) examines the extent to which PEPFAR policies and procedures adhere to established general principles for the evaluation of U.S. government programs.

To address these objectives, we reviewed the American Evaluation Association's (AEA) *An Evaluation Roadmap for a More Effective Government* (AEA Roadmap)[5] as well as policies and guidance developed by the Department of State (State), State's Office of the U.S. Global AIDS Coordinator (OGAC), the Department of Health and Human Services' (HHS) Centers for Disease Control and Prevention (CDC), and the U.S. Agency for International Development (USAID). We conducted interviews with officials at OGAC, USAID, and CDC. We also surveyed CDC and USAID headquarters officials as well as CDC and USAID officials in the 31 countries and 3 regions that had PEPFAR annual operational plans in fiscal year 2010[6] about which of their PEPFAR-funded activities operating in fiscal years 2008 through 2010 had ongoing or completed evaluations. In addition, we obtained electronic copies of

---

[4]The Consolidated Appropriations Act directed GAO to review PEPFAR "results monitoring activities," among other things. See Pub. L. No. 110-161, § 668(d), 121 Stat. 1844, 2353 (2007). The 2008 Leadership Act directed GAO to provide a report including "a description and assessment of the monitoring and evaluation practices and policies in place" for U.S. bilateral global HIV/AIDS programs, among other things. See Pub. L. No. 110-293, § 101(d). In response to these directives, we also issued *President's Emergency Plan for AIDS Relief: Program Planning and Reporting* (GAO-11-785) in July 2011. A list of related GAO products, including past work conducted in response to these congressional mandates, is provided at the end of this report.

[5]The American Evaluation Association, an international professional association for evaluators of programs, products, personnel, and policies, developed general principles for the work of professionals in everyday practice and to inform evaluation clients and the general public of expectations for ethical behavior. For more information, see American Evaluation Association, *An Evaluation Roadmap for a More Effective Government* (Washington, D.C.: 2010), accessed March 31, 2012, http://www.eval.org/Publications/GuidingPrinciples.asp.

[6]The 31 countries were Angola, Botswana, Cambodia, China, Côte d'Ivoire, Democratic Republic of the Congo, Dominican Republic, Ethiopia, Ghana, Guyana, Haiti, India, Indonesia, Kenya, Lesotho, Malawi, Mozambique, Namibia, Nigeria, Russia, Rwanda, South Africa, Sudan, Swaziland, Tanzania, Thailand, Uganda, Ukraine, Vietnam, Zambia, and Zimbabwe. The 3 regions were the Caribbean, Central America, and Central Asia.

completed evaluations for programs operating during this time period from CDC and USAID officials at headquarters and in the PEPFAR countries and regions. Using a standard assessment tool, we systematically assessed the level of support for findings, conclusions, and recommendations in samples of these evaluations, as indicated by the degree to which they were conducted in adherence with selected common evaluation standards. We assessed judgmental samples of evaluations submitted by OGAC and by CDC and USAID headquarters. We assessed a randomly selected sample of the evaluations submitted by PEPFAR country and regional teams, in order to generalize our assessment results to all of the submitted evaluations. Finally, we assessed State, OGAC, CDC, and USAID policies and practices against selected general principles of evaluation defined in the AEA Roadmap. (See app. I for a detailed description of our objectives, scope, and methodology.)

We conducted this performance audit from October 2011 to May 2012 in accordance with generally accepted government auditing standards. Those standards require that we plan and perform the audit to obtain sufficient, appropriate evidence to provide a reasonable basis for our findings and conclusions based on our audit objectives. We believe that the evidence obtained provides a reasonable basis for our findings and conclusions based on our audit objectives.

Background

OGAC establishes overall PEPFAR policy and program strategies and coordinates PEPFAR program activities. In addition, OGAC allocates PEPFAR resources from the Global Health and Child Survival account to PEPFAR implementing agencies, primarily CDC and USAID.[7] The agencies execute PEPFAR program activities through agency headquarters offices[8] and interagency teams consisting of PEPFAR implementing agency officials in the countries and regions with PEPFAR-funded programs (PEPFAR country and regional teams). OGAC

---

[7]Other PEPFAR implementing agencies are the Departments of State, Defense, Labor, and Commerce and the Peace Corps. Additional HHS offices and agencies receiving PEPFAR resources are the Office of Global Affairs, the Food and Drug Administration, the Health Resources and Services Administration, the National Institutes of Health, and the Substance Abuse and Mental Health Services Administration.

[8]CDC's Division of Global HIV/AIDS (DGHA) and USAID's Office of HIV/AIDS (OHA) have responsibility for coordinating PEPFAR program implementation.

coordinates these activities through its approval of operational plans, which serve as annual work plans and document planned investments in, and the anticipated results of, HIV/AIDS-related programs. OGAC provides annual guidance on how to develop and submit operational plans.

In fiscal years 2009 through 2011, OGAC approved operational plans representing $11.7 billion in PEPFAR program activities. These activities fall primarily in three broad program areas—prevention, treatment, and care—and 18 related program areas.[9] Program activities aimed at preventing HIV infection and at treating those infected each represented about 30 percent of approved PEPFAR funding, while activities aimed at caring for AIDS patients represented about 20 percent. The remaining approximately 20 percent funded a variety of other program areas, such as health systems strengthening and building laboratory infrastructure. Figure 1 summarizes approved funding for these program areas in fiscal years 2009 through 2011.

---

[9]Prevention-related program areas are mother-to-child transmission, abstinence/be faithful, other sexual prevention, blood safety, injection safety, medical male circumcision, prevention among injecting and noninjecting drug users, and testing and counseling. Treatment-related program areas are antiretroviral drugs, adult treatment, and pediatric treatment. Care-related program areas are adult care and support, pediatric care and support, orphans and vulnerable children, and tuberculosis/HIV. Other program areas are laboratory infrastructure, strategic information, and health systems strengthening.

Figure 1: Approved Funding for PEPFAR Prevention, Treatment, Care, and Other Program Areas, Fiscal Years 2009 through 2011

Program area

Prevention

| $936.5 | $567.0 | $819.5 | | | | | $628.5 | **Total $3,473.9 (29.7%)** |

Prevention of mother-to-child transmission (8.0%)

Abstinence/ be faithful (4.9%)

Other sexual prevention (7.0%)

$167.3 Blood safety (1.4%)

$71.4 Injection safety (0.6%)

$69.6 Prevention among injecting and non-injecting drug users (0.6%)

$214.1 Medical male circumcision (1.8%)

Testing and counseling (5.4%)

Care

| $975.3 | | $1,011.3 | $439.5 | **Total $2,585.8 (22.1%)** |

Adult care and support (8.3%)

$159.7 Pediatric care and support (1.4%)

Orphans and vulnerable children (8.7%)

TB/HIV (3.8%)

Treatment

| $1,125.5 | $2,016.3 | $319.2 | **Total $3,461.0 (29.6%)** |

Antiretroviral drugs (9.6%)

Adult treatment (17.2%)

Pediatric treatment (2.7%)

Other

| $610.3 | $580.0 | $983.1 | **Total $2,173.4 (18.6%)** |

Laboratory infrastructure (5.2%)

Strategic information (5.0%)

Health systems strengthening (8.4%)

0   500   1,000   1,500   2,000   2,500   3,000   3,500   4,000

Dollars in millions

PEPFAR approved funding for prevention, treatment, care, and other programs, FY 2009-2011: $11.7 billion

Source: GAO analysis of OGAC data reported in FY 2009-2011 PEPFAR operational places.

Note: Numbers do not always add to totals because of rounding. These OGAC data were reported in PEPFAR operational plans for fiscal years 2009 through 2011.

To carry out activities in these program areas, CDC and USAID use implementing mechanisms—grants, cooperative agreements, and contracts—with a variety of implementing partners.[10] These partners include partner country governments, nongovernmental and international organizations, and academic institutions. CDC and USAID used more than 3,000 implementing mechanisms in fiscal years 2008 through 2010.

CDC and USAID offices employ a wide variety of individuals and organizations to conduct PEPFAR evaluations, including implementing agency officials, consultants, and academic institutions as well as partner government organizations and implementing partners. Evaluation teams sometimes comprise representatives from several of these organizations. OGAC coordinates, and PEPFAR implementing agencies also engage in, several related activities that support evaluation, such as oversight of implementing partners,[11] routine performance planning and reporting,[12] biological and behavioral health surveillance,[13] baseline studies and

---

[10]According to OGAC guidance, an implementing mechanism is a grant, cooperative agreement, or contract in which a discrete dollar amount is passed through a prime implementing partner and for which the prime implementing partner is held fiscally accountable.

[11]See GAO, *President's Emergency Plan for AIDS Relief: Partner Selection and Oversight Follow Accepted Practices but Would Benefit from Enhanced Planning and Accountability*, GAO-09-666 (Washington, D.C.: July 15, 2009).

[12]See GAO, *President's Emergency Plan for AIDS Relief: Program Planning and Reporting*, GAO-11-785 (Washington, D.C.: July 29, 2011).

[13]Public health surveillance is the continuous, systematic collection, analysis, and interpretation of health-related data needed for the planning, implementation, and evaluation of public health programs. Surveillance can serve as an early warning system for impending public health emergencies; document the impact of an intervention, or track progress toward specified goals; and monitor and clarify the epidemiology of health problems, to allow priorities to be set and to inform public health policy and strategies.

needs assessments, and development of health management information systems.[14]

PEPFAR evaluations are subject to common evaluation standards defined in various agency-specific and governmentwide guidance. This guidance includes CDC's Framework for Program Evaluation in Public Health[15] and USAID's evaluation policy[16] and Automated Directives System guidance.[17] In addition, GAO published guidance on designing evaluations and assessing social program impact evaluations.[18]

Also, in September 2010, the AEA published a framework to guide the development and implementation of federal agency evaluation programs and policies. The framework offers a set of general principles intended to

---

[14]In March 2011, in an article published in the *Journal of Acquired Immune Deficiency Syndromes*, the U.S. Global AIDS Coordinator and other senior PEPFAR officials wrote that given PEPFAR's emergency response during its first 5 years, "state-of-the-art monitoring, evaluation, and research methodologies were not fully integrated or systematically performed." As such, for PEPFAR's second 5 years, to demonstrate value and impact in resource-constrained environments, PEPFAR adopted an "implementation science" framework, which, in turn, includes monitoring and evaluation, operations research, and impact evaluation as its main components. See "Implementation Science for the U.S. President's Emergency Plan for AIDS Relief (PEPFAR)," *Journal of Acquired Immune Deficiency Syndromes*, vol. 56, no. 3 (March 1, 2011).

[15]Department of Health and Human Services, Centers for Disease Control and Prevention, "Framework for Program Evaluation in Public Health," *Morbidity and Mortality Weekly Report: Recommendations and Reports*, vol. 48, no. RR-11 (September 1999), accessed May 23, 2012, http://www.cdc.gov/eval/framework/index.htm.

[16]U.S. Agency for International Development, Bureau for Policy, Planning, and Learning, Office of Learning, Evaluation, and Research, *Evaluation: Learning from Experience, USAID Evaluation Policy* (Washington, D.C.: January 2011), accessed May 23, 2012, http://www.usaid.gov/evaluation/USAIDEvaluationPolicy.pdf.

[17]U.S. Agency for International Development, "USAID Evaluation Policy: Automated Directives System, Chapter 203: Assessing and Learning" (2010). The Automated Directives System is USAID's directives management program. Agency policy directives, required procedures, and helpful, optional material are drafted, cleared, and issued through this system. Agency employees must adhere to these policy directives and required procedures.

[18]GAO, *Designing Evaluations: 2012 Revision*, GAO-12-208G (Washington, D.C.: January 2012). This document addresses the logic of program evaluation designs, describes different types of evaluations and the process for designing them, and highlights issues related to overall evaluation quality. Further, it updates GAO/PEMD-10.1.4 (*Designing Evaluations*, March 1991), which we used to develop our evaluation assessment tool. For more information, see appendix I.

facilitate the integration of evaluation activities with program management. These principles include developing evaluation policies and procedures; developing evaluation plans; ensuring independence of evaluators in designing, conducting, and determining findings of their evaluations; ensuring professional competence of evaluators; and disseminating evaluation results publicly and in a timely fashion.[19]

PEPFAR Agencies Have Evaluated a Broad Range of PEPFAR Programs, but Results Are Not Fully Supported in Many Evaluations

OGAC, CDC, and USAID managed and conducted evaluations of a wide variety of PEPFAR programs that were ongoing during fiscal years 2008 through 2010. However, we found that many of these evaluations—particularly evaluations managed by PEPFAR country and regional teams—did not consistently adhere to common evaluation standards, in many cases calling into question the evaluations' support for their findings, conclusions, and recommendations.

OGAC, CDC, and USAID Evaluated a Broad Range of Programs

OGAC, CDC, and USAID provided 496 evaluations addressing programs ongoing during fiscal years 2008 to 2010 in all PEPFAR program areas relating to HIV/AIDS treatment, prevention, and care. Of these 496 evaluations, 18 were public health evaluations (PHE), managed by OGAC; 42 were program evaluations provided by CDC and USAID headquarters officials; and 436 were program evaluations provided by CDC and USAID country and regional team officials. (For more information about these evaluations, see app. III.)

- **OGAC-managed evaluations.** OGAC provided 18 PHEs that CDC and USAID had completed as of November 2011 under an OGAC-managed approval, implementation review, and reporting process. The completed PHEs addressed the following program areas: prevention of mother-to-child transmission, testing and counseling, adult care and support, adult treatment, sexual prevention, and

---

[19]Two additional AEA Roadmap principles that we did not address in this report relate to integrating evaluation into planning, developing, and managing programs and providing stable, continuous funding for evaluation.

pediatric care and support.[20] In addition, OGAC indicated that 82 other PHEs had been initiated as of November 2011. According to OGAC, PHEs are intended to assess the effectiveness and impact of PEPFAR programs; compare evidence-based program models in complex health, social, and economic contexts; and address operational questions related to program implementation within existing and developing health systems infrastructures. OGAC guidance states that these evaluations focus on strategies to increase program efficiency and impact to guide program development and inform the public, using rigorous quantitative or qualitative methods that permit broad generalization. For all PHEs, OGAC requires PEPFAR country and regional teams to submit evaluation concepts or protocols for approval by an interagency subcommittee[21] and requires periodic progress and closeout reports.

- **CDC and USAID headquarters-managed evaluations.** CDC headquarters officials provided 20 evaluations in the following program areas: blood safety, injection safety, adult treatment, pediatric treatment, and strategic information. USAID headquarters officials provided 22 evaluations in the following program areas: abstinence/be faithful, sexual prevention, orphans and vulnerable children, strategic information, and health systems strengthening programs. Four CDC and USAID headquarters evaluations addressed more than one program area.

- **Country and regional team-managed evaluations.** CDC and USAID officials representing 31 PEPFAR country and 3 regional teams provided a total of 436 evaluations; CDC officials provided 185 evaluations, and USAID officials provided 251 evaluations. The evaluations addressed 18 program areas related to PEPFAR prevention, treatment, and care, with about one-fifth of the evaluations addressing activities in more than one program area (see fig. 2). CDC

---

[20] According to a journal article written by OGAC and other officials, PHEs have been relatively limited in number and disparate in the range of research questions. See Padian et al., "Implementation Science for the U.S. President's Emergency Plan for AIDS Relief (PEPFAR)."

[21] PEPFAR's public health evaluation interagency subcommittee oversees PEPFAR policies and procedures for proposing, approving, and disseminating the results of PEPFAR public health evaluations. OGAC's Office of Research and Science, established in October 2011, coordinates the work of the PHE subcommittee and their interactions with implementing agencies, country teams, and other stakeholders.

GAO-12-673 PEPFAR Evaluations

and USAID officials also provided copies of evaluation protocols and statements of work, indicating that additional evaluations had been initiated. Further, based on our analysis of a randomly selected sample of 78 evaluations,[22] we estimate that 51 percent of the evaluations used qualitative methods, 35 percent used quantitative methods, and 14 percent used a mix of quantitative and qualitative methods.[23] In addition, evaluations provided by USAID tended to employ qualitative methods (32 of 48 evaluations), while those provided by CDC tended to use quantitative methods (20 of 30 evaluations). (See app. III for additional results of our analysis.)

---

[22]We drew a probability sample of 84 of 436 evaluations submitted by CDC and USAID officials in 31 PEPFAR countries and 3 regions. Six cases were found to be out of scope, resulting in a sample of 78. Results based on random probability samples are subject to sampling error. The sample we drew for our survey is only one of a large number of samples we might have drawn. Because different samples could have provided different estimates, we express our confidence in the precision of our particular sample results as a 95 percent confidence interval. This is the interval that would contain the actual population values for 95 percent of the samples we could have drawn. The margin of error associated with proportion estimates is no more than plus or minus 11 percentage points at the 95 percent level of confidence. The margin of error for totals is not more than 44 evaluations.

[23]Qualitative methods include collecting data through interviews, focus groups, document or literature reviews, and observation, and analyzing data by discerning, examining, comparing, and contrasting meaningful patterns or themes in qualitative data. Quantitative methods typically involve collecting quantifiable information through probability sampling and using various forms of statistical analysis to generalize results. Evaluations using mixed methods employ a combination of qualitative and quantitative data collection and analysis techniques. See appendix III for more information.

Figure 2: Program Evaluations Provided by PEPFAR Country and Regional Teams, by PEPFAR Program Area

Program area

Prevention — Total 82 evaluations (18.8%)
- 19 — Prevention of mother-to-child transmission (4.4%)
- 10 — Abstinence/be faithful (2.3%)
- 29 — Other sexual prevention (6.7%)
- 6 — Blood safety (1.4%)
- 4 — Injection safety (0.9%)
- 1 — Medical male circumcision (0.2%)
- 4 — Prevention among injecting and non-injecting drug users (0.9%)
- 9 — Testing and counseling (2.1%)

Care — Total 102 evaluations (23.4%)
- 14 — Adult care and support (3.2%)
- 3 — Pediatric care and support (0.7%)
- 63 — Orphans and vulnerable children (14.4%)
- 22 — TB/HIV (5.0%)

Treatment — Total 68 evaluations (15.6%)
- 7 — Antiretroviral drugs (1.6%)
- 49 — Adult treatment (11.2%)
- 12 — Pediatric treatment (2.8%)

Other — Total 93 evaluations (21.3%)
- 12 — Laboratory infrastructure (2.8%)
- 29 — Strategic information (6.7%)
- 52 — Health systems strengthening (11.9%)

More than one program area — Total 91 evaluations (20.9%)

Number of evaluations: 0, 20, 40, 60, 80, 100, 120

Total number of evaluations: 436

Source: GAO analysis of evaluations submitted by 31 country and 3 regional PEPFAR teams.

Note: Percentages do not always add to totals because of rounding. We initially identified 436 evaluations provided by CDC and USAID officials in 31 PEPFAR country and 3 regional teams. After examining a sample of 84 evaluations drawn from these 436 evaluations, we determined that a subset of these were outside the scope of our review. However, this figure presents counts by program area for all 436 evaluations. See appendix I for more information.

Findings, Conclusions, and Recommendations Are Not Fully Supported in Many Evaluations

Our assessments of judgmental and randomly selected samples of PEPFAR evaluations indicate that many—particularly those managed by PEPFAR country and regional teams—contain findings, conclusions, and recommendations that are not fully supported. To determine the extent to which these elements are supported, we synthesized our assessments of the extent to which evaluations generally adhered to several common evaluation standards defined in guidance issued by CDC, USAID, and GAO. Specifically, we considered whether the evaluations describe the program to be evaluated and its objectives, the purpose of the evaluation, and the criteria used to reach conclusions about the achievement of the program's objectives. We also considered the extent to which evaluations incorporate appropriate designs, sample selection methods, measures, and data collection and analysis methods.

All OGAC-managed PHEs that we reviewed generally adhered to these standards and thus their findings, conclusions, and recommendations were fully supported. We found similar results for most CDC and USAID headquarters' program evaluations we reviewed. However, PEPFAR country and regional teams' evaluations did not consistently adhere to common evaluation standards, and thus, in most cases, their findings, conclusions, and recommendations were not fully supported.

OGAC-managed evaluations. Our assessment of seven OGAC-managed PEPFAR PHEs indicates that they all generally adhered to common evaluation standards, and thus their findings, conclusions, and recommendations were fully supported.[24] All of the evaluations that we reviewed identified program and evaluation objectives and used appropriate measures, and most used appropriate evaluation designs and data collection and analysis methods. Three of the evaluations employed fully appropriate sampling methods. Table 1 summarizes our assessments of these evaluations.

[24]From the 18 completed PHEs submitted by OGAC, we selected a judgmental sample of 7 evaluations based on the type of program (e.g., prevention, treatment, care, or other) evaluated as well as the country or countries addressed by each evaluation. Because this is a judgmental sample, results should not be used to make inferences about all evaluations managed by OGAC; however, the PHEs selected represent a mix of the types of evaluations managed by OGAC. See appendix I for more information.

Table 1: Level of Support for Evaluation Findings, Conclusions, and Recommendations in Selected OGAC-Managed Public Health Evaluations, as Indicated by Adherence to Common Evaluation Standards

	GAO assessments (n=7)		
	Yes	Partial	No
Findings, conclusions, and recommendations appear to be fully supported[a]	7	0	0
Common evaluation standards			
Evaluation identifies program and evaluation objectives	7	0	0
Evaluation specifies why evaluation is needed	7	0	0
Evaluation identifies evaluation criteria	5	2	0
Evaluation design appears to be appropriate	5	2	0
Participant/sample selection methods and sample size appear to be generally appropriate	3	4	0
Measures used for this evaluation appear to be appropriate	7	0	0
Data collection and analysis methods appear to be appropriate	6	1	0

Source: GAO analysis.

[a]Overall determinations are based on synthesis—but not tally—of assessments of adherence to common evaluation standards listed in this table. See appendix I for more information.

CDC and USAID headquarters-managed evaluations. Our assessment of 15 CDC and USAID headquarters-managed evaluations indicates that most generally adhere to common evaluation standards.[25] As a result, we found that findings, conclusions, and recommendations were fully supported in 9 evaluations and partially supported in 6 evaluations. Most of the evaluations employed appropriate evaluation designs, measures, and data collection and analysis methods. However, 7 evaluations did not fully identify the evaluation criteria, and 8 did not employ fully appropriate sampling methods. Table 2 summarizes our assessments of these evaluations.

---

[25]From the 42 evaluations we received from CDC and USAID headquarters (20 from CDC, 22 from USAID), we selected a judgmental sample of 15 evaluations (7 from CDC, 8 from USAID) based on the type of program (e.g., prevention, treatment, care, or other) evaluated as well as the country or countries addressed by each evaluation. Because this is a judgmental sample, results should not be used to make inferences about all evaluations managed by CDC and USAID headquarters. However, they represent a mix of the types of evaluations managed by CDC and USAID headquarters. See appendix I for more information.

Table 2: Level of Support for Evaluation Findings, Conclusions, and Recommendations in Selected CDC and USAID Headquarters-Managed Evaluations, as Indicated by Adherence to Common Evaluation Standards

	GAO assessments (n=15)		
	Yes	Partial	No
Findings, conclusions, and recommendations appear to be fully supported[a]	9	6	0
Common evaluation standards			
Evaluation identifies program and evaluation objectives	13	2	0
Evaluation specifies why the evaluation is needed	14	0	1
Evaluation identifies evaluation criteria	8	4	3
Evaluation design appears to be appropriate	10	4	1
Participant/sample selection methods and sample size appear to be generally appropriate	7	6	2
Measures used for this evaluation appear to be appropriate	10	2	3
Data collection and analysis methods appear to be appropriate	12	2	1

Source: GAO analysis.

[a]Overall determinations are based on synthesis—but not tally—of assessments of adherence to common evaluation standards listed in this table. See appendix I for more information.

Country and regional team-managed evaluations. We found that evaluations managed by country and regional teams, which make up the bulk of all PEPFAR program evaluations, did not consistently adhere to common evaluation standards. Based on our analysis of a randomly selected sample of country and regional team evaluations, we estimate that findings, conclusions, and recommendations were fully supported in 41 percent of all evaluations provided to us by country and regional teams, partially supported in 44 percent of these evaluations, and not supported in 15 percent of these evaluations.[26] We estimate that 24

---

[26]We drew a probability sample of 84 of 436 evaluations submitted by CDC and USAID officials in 31 PEPFAR countries and 3 regions. Six cases were found to be out of scope, resulting in a sample of 78. Results based on random probability samples are subject to sampling error. The sample we drew for our survey is only one of a large number of samples we might have drawn. Because different samples could have provided different estimates, we express our confidence in the precision of our particular sample results as a 95 percent confidence interval. This is the interval that would contain the actual population values for 95 percent of the samples we could have drawn. The margin of error associated with proportion estimates is no more than plus or minus 11 percentage points at the 95 percent level of confidence. The margin of error for totals is not more than 44 evaluations.

percent of these evaluations did not identify any evaluation criteria, and more than half did not employ evaluation designs, sampling methods, measures, or data collection and analysis methods that were fully appropriate.[27] For example, an evaluation of activities for providing care to orphans and vulnerable children drew conclusions about results and made recommendations, based almost exclusively on favorable anecdotal information collected from selected program participants and beneficiaries. As a result, the objectivity and credibility of these evaluations' findings, conclusions, and recommendations are in question. Table 3 summarizes our assessments of these evaluations.

---

[27]A June 2011 assessment of 56 USAID evaluations—including 8 evaluations of programs funded at least in part through PEPFAR—found that 41 of the evaluations used appropriate data collection methods, while 15 evaluations used data collection methods that were deemed to be partially or somewhat appropriate. See Office of the Director of U.S. Foreign Assistance, *A Meta Evaluation of Foreign Assistance Evaluations* (Washington, D.C.: June 2011), accessed October 2011, http://pdf.usaid.gov/pdf_docs/PCAAC273.pdf.

Table 3: Estimated Extent to Which Country and Regional Teams' Evaluations Contained Fully Supported Findings, Conclusions, and Recommendations, as Measured by Adherence to Common Evaluation Standards

	GAO assessments (n=436)			
	Yes	Partial	No	Not applicable
Findings, conclusions, and recommendations appear to be fully supported[a]	179 (41 percent)	190 (44 percent)	67 (15 percent)	0 (0 percent)
Common evaluation standards				
Evaluation identifies program and evaluation objectives	363 (83 percent)	73 (17 percent)	0 (0 percent)	0 (0 percent)
Evaluation specifies why the evaluation is needed	375 (86 percent)	56 (13 percent)	6 (1 percent)	0 (0 percent)
Evaluation identifies evaluation criteria	224 (51 percent)	106 (24 percent)	106 (24 percent)	0 (0 percent)
Evaluation design appears to be appropriate	212 (49 percent)	184 (42 percent)	39 (9 percent)	0 (0 percent)
Participant/sample selection methods and sample size appear to be generally appropriate	168 (38 percent)	123 (28 percent)	117 (27 percent)	28 (6 percent)
Measures used for this evaluation appear to be appropriate	196 (45 percent)	140 (32 percent)	84 (19 percent)	17 (4 percent)
Data collection and analysis methods appear to be appropriate	134 (31 percent)	229 (53 percent)	73 (17 percent)	0 (0 percent)

Source: GAO analysis.

[a]Overall determinations are based on synthesis—but not tally—of assessments of adherence to common evaluation standards listed in this table. See app. I for more information.

Notes: Numbers and percentages are based on analysis of a randomly selected sample of evaluations. The margin of error associated with proportion estimates is no more than plus or minus 11 percentage points at the 95 percent level of confidence. The margin of error for totals is not more than 44 evaluations. Numbers do not always add to totals because of rounding. See appendices I and III for more information about these assessments.

Further analysis of the results of our assessments showed that evaluations using qualitative methods were more likely to contain results that were partially supported or not supported than evaluations using quantitative methods. (See app. III for additional results of our analysis.)

PEPFAR Policies and Procedures Do Not Fully Adhere to AEA Evaluation Principles Relating to Planning, Independence, and Dissemination

State, OGAC, CDC, and USAID have developed policies and procedures that apply to evaluations of PEPFAR programs, as called for in the AEA Roadmap. However, they have not fully adhered to other AEA Roadmap principles regarding evaluation planning, independence and competence of evaluators, and dissemination of evaluation results. First, OGAC has not developed PEPFAR evaluation plans at the program level or required the development of such plans in individual countries and regions, limiting its own ability to ensure that evaluation resources are appropriately targeted. Second, State, OGAC, CDC, and USAID guidance does not specify how to document the independence and competency of evaluators, and almost half of the evaluations we reviewed did not provide sufficient information to fully determine whether evaluators were free of conflicts of interest. Finally, not all evaluation reports are available online, thus limiting their accessibility and usefulness to PEPFAR decision makers and other stakeholders.

State, OGAC, and PEPFAR Implementing Agencies Have Issued Evaluation Policies and Procedures

In accordance with AEA principles, State, OGAC, CDC, and USAID have issued policies and procedures that are applicable to PEPFAR program evaluation.[28]

- **State evaluation policy.** In February 2012, State's Bureau of Resource Management issued an evaluation policy that applies to all State bureaus and OGAC.[29] The policy provides a framework for implementing evaluations of State's various programs and projects and encourages evaluations for programs and projects at all funding levels.

---

[28]The AEA Roadmap advises agencies to publish policies and procedures for conducting evaluations within their purview. These policies and procedures should provide guidance to evaluators, identifying the kinds of evaluations to be performed and defining administrative steps for developing evaluation plans, setting priorities, ensuring evaluation product quality and independence, and publishing evaluation reports.

[29] State's evaluation policy requires evaluation of all large programs, projects, and activities at least once in their lifetime or every 5 years, whichever is less. Further, the policy notes that some State bureaus and OGAC do not directly implement projects or programs and, instead, provide funds to other agencies or operating units. In these cases, State bureaus and OGAC are expected to ensure that implementing organizations carry out evaluations of programs, projects, and activities consistent with State policy. For more information see State, *Department of State Program Evaluation Policy* (Washington, D.C.: Feb. 23, 2012), accessed March 31, 2012, http://www.state.gov/s/d/rm/rls/evaluation/2012/184556.htm.

- **OGAC operational plan guidance.** According to OGAC officials, OGAC generally has deferred to implementing agency policies. OGAC also issues annual guidance to PEPFAR implementing agencies for preparation of their operational plans. OGAC's fiscal year 2012 operational plan guidance to PEPFAR country and regional teams, issued in August 2011, addresses some elements of evaluation. The guidance differentiates three types of evaluation and research: basic program evaluation, which focuses on descriptive and normative evaluation questions; operations research, which focuses on program delivery and optimal allocation of resources; and impact evaluation, which measures the change in an outcome attributable to a particular program.[30]

- **CDC evaluation framework.** In September 1999, the Program Evaluation Unit at CDC's Office of the Associate Director for Program issued an evaluation framework for CDC programs.[31] The framework summarizes essential elements of program evaluation, clarifies program evaluation steps, and reviews standards for effective program evaluation, among other things. According to CDC's Chief Evaluation Officer, as of May 2012, CDC plans to issue evaluation guidelines and recommendations as well as additional guidance for using the evaluation framework.

- **USAID evaluation policy.** In January 2011, USAID's Bureau for Policy, Planning, and Learning revised evaluation policy to supplement existing evaluation guidance in USAID's Automated Directive System.[32] According to USAID, this revised policy was intended to address a decline in the quantity and quality of evaluation practice within the agency in the recent past. The policy clarifies for USAID staff, partners, and stakeholders the purposes of evaluation; the types of evaluations that are required and recommended; and

---

[30]For current guidance, see *The President's Emergency Plan for AIDS Relief, FY 2012 Technical Considerations Provided by PEPFAR Technical Working Groups for FY 2012 COPs and ROPs* (Washington, D.C.: 2011), accessed March 31, 2012, http://www.pepfar.gov/documents/organization/169737.pdf.

[31]Department of Health and Human Services, Centers for Disease Control and Prevention, "Framework for Program Evaluation in Public Health." CDC's Program Evaluation Unit sets standards and expectations for evaluation and provides tools, technical assistance, and resources to enhance CDC's evaluation efforts.

[32]USAID, Bureau for Policy, Planning, and Learning, Office of Learning, Evaluation, and Research, *Evaluation: Learning from Experience, USAID Evaluation Policy.*

USAID's approach for conducting, disseminating, and using evaluations. Among other things, the policy sets forth the purposes of evaluation, the roles and responsibilities of USAID operating units, and evaluation requirements and practices for all USAID programs and projects. The policy requires all USAID operating units to consult with program office experts to ensure that scopes of work for external evaluations meet evaluation standards. The policy also states that operating units, in collaboration with the program office, must ensure that evaluation draft reports are assessed for quality by management and through an in-house peer technical review.[33]

PEPFAR Lacks Evaluation Plans

OGAC has not yet developed a program-level PEPFAR evaluation plan or required implementing agencies or country and regional teams to develop evaluation plans as called for by the AEA Roadmap.[34]

- **OGAC.** State's recently issued evaluation policy requires that each State bureau, including OGAC, develop and submit a bureauwide evaluation plan that encompasses major policy initiatives and new programs as well as existing programs and projects. According to a senior OGAC official, at the time of our review, OGAC was discussing with State's Bureau of Resource Management how it will comply with this new requirement.

- **CDC and USAID headquarters.** OGAC defers to implementing agencies to plan evaluations of their headquarters-managed PEPFAR program activities, but CDC and USAID have not developed evaluation plans for such activities included in recent headquarters operational plans. OGAC's 2011 guidance for developing the headquarters operational plan requires a plan for technical area

---

[33]USAID reported in February 2012 that it had taken several steps to implement the new evaluation policy, including training USAID staff in evaluation and establishing an evaluation point of contact in every USAID field mission. USAID's Office of HIV/AIDS provides technical assistance, training, and other support to USAID mission officials and other implementing partners responsible for implementing PEPFAR programs. See USAID. *Evaluation Policy: Year One, First Annual Report and Plan for 2012 and 2013* (Washington, D.C.: February 2012), accessed March 31, 2012, http://www.usaid.gov/evaluation/USAIDEvaluationPolicy-YearOne.pdf.

[34]The AEA Roadmap states that major program components should prepare annual and multiyear evaluation plans, taking into account the need for evaluation results to inform program budgeting, reauthorization, strategic planning, program development and management, and questions of program effectiveness.

program priorities but does not address evaluation planning. Similarly, the fiscal year 2012 guidance does not include a requirement for an evaluation plan.

- **Country and regional teams.** OGAC defers to PEPFAR country and regional teams to plan evaluations of their program activities, but does not require that the teams develop and submit annual evaluation plans. OGAC's 2011 guidance on developing country and regional operational plans urges country and regional teams to prioritize program evaluation in order to make PEPFAR programs more effective and sustainable. In addition, OGAC's fiscal year 2012 guidance calls for country and regional teams to address monitoring and evaluation in describing individual implementing partners' activities. However, neither the 2011 guidance nor the 2012 guidance instructs all country teams to develop evaluation plans.[35] We reviewed PEPFAR country and regional operational plans for fiscal year 2011 and found that they did not include evaluation plans.[36] Instead, these documents generally included (1) descriptions of ongoing or planned evaluations and related activities (e.g., surveillance) in program area narrative summaries and (2) descriptions of monitoring and evaluation activities in implementing partner activity narratives.

In our analysis of information provided by country and regional teams, as well as CDC and USAID headquarters, we did not detect an evaluation rationale or strategy. Based on responses to our survey of CDC and

---

[35]An addendum to OGAC's fiscal year 2012 operational plan guidance, issued in November 2011, states that some country teams could submit a country implementation science strategy, as part of a pilot initiative, which would include descriptions of monitoring and evaluation activities, current knowledge gaps, reference to implementation science strategies and priorities, descriptions of ongoing evaluations, and implementation science and priorities for the coming year. OGAC officials further clarified that the pilot initiative would begin in fiscal year 2013. At the time of our review, the fiscal year 2012 country and regional operational plans had not yet been approved, and thus it is too early to determine how country and regional teams have implemented this new guidance.

[36]We reviewed 11 country operational plans and 2 regional operational plans for fiscal year 2011.

USAID officials in 31 PEPFAR country and 3 regional teams,[37] we calculated that evaluations had been conducted or were ongoing for about one-third of these countries' program activities in fiscal years 2008 through 2010. In addition, based on these officials' responses, we found similar percentages of ongoing and completed evaluations across the broad program areas of prevention, treatment, and care.[38] We also analyzed CDC and USAID headquarters officials' responses to our survey and found that evaluations had been conducted or were ongoing for about half of the PEPFAR program activities managed by agencies' headquarters and implemented during fiscal years 2008 to 2010.[39] However, we found no relationships between the percentages of program activities with ongoing or completed evaluations and budgets at the country, program area (i.e., prevention, treatment, or care), or program activity levels.

Evaluator Independence and Qualifications Are Not Consistently Documented

State, CDC, and USAID policies and procedures address the independence of evaluators but do not consistently require that evaluation reports identify the evaluation team or address whether there are any potential conflicts of interest.[40] In addition, some agency policies and procedures address the need to ensure that evaluators have appropriate

---

[37]We sent a total of 67 questionnaires to CDC and USAID officials in the 31 PEPFAR countries and 3 PEPFAR regions that were required to submit PEPFAR country or regional operational plans in fiscal year 2010. The questionnaires took form as spreadsheets listing each agency's PEPFAR implementing mechanisms—a proxy for program activity—from fiscal years 2008 through 2010 and prompted officials to indicate whether each implementing mechanism had an ongoing or completed evaluation. See app. I for more information.

[38]CDC and USAID officials responding to our survey also indicated that a higher percentage of program activities had evaluations that were ongoing for programs starting in later years, that some programs at the time of our survey were not sufficiently completed for evaluation, and that evaluations were planned for later in the program life cycle.

[39]CDC and USAID officials reported roughly the same percentages of PEPFAR programs with ongoing or completed evaluations. CDC officials more frequently reported that evaluations were broader than individual program activities, compared to USAID officials.

[40]According to the AEA Roadmap, agencies should safeguard the independence of evaluators in the design and performance of evaluations and in presentation of the results. Agencies should also promote objectivity in examining program operations and impact.

qualifications, but none require that evaluations document those qualifications or certify that they are adequate.[41]

- **State.** State's recently issued evaluation policy addresses evaluator independence and integrity, stating that evaluators should be free from program managers and not subject to their influence. This policy does not address evaluator qualifications.

- **OGAC.** OGAC's operational plan guidance to country and regional teams does not address the independence or professional qualifications of evaluators. According to OGAC officials, OGAC defers to implementing agency evaluation policies.

- **CDC.** CDC's evaluation framework addresses the need to assemble an evaluation team with the needed competencies, highlighting the importance of ensuring that evaluators have no particular stake in the results of the evaluation. The CDC evaluation framework also discusses appropriate ways to assemble an evaluation team.

- **USAID.** USAID's evaluation policy recommends that most evaluations be external and requires a disclosure of conflicts of interest for all evaluation team members. In addition, USAID's evaluation policy requires that evaluation-related competencies be included in staffing selection policies.

Our analysis of a randomly selected sample of evaluations submitted by 31 PEPFAR country and 3 regional teams found that the evaluations often did not address whether evaluators have potential conflicts of interest, as called for by the AEA Roadmap. We estimate that 27 percent of the evaluations fully addressed potential conflicts of interest, 59 percent partially addressed the issue, and 14 percent did not address the issue. In addition, while we were unable to determine whether potential conflicts of interest existed with the information provided in some of the evaluation reports, it appeared that there were evaluations in which potential conflicts of interest existed but were not addressed. For example, one evaluation report, relating to strengthening a partner country's nongovernmental HIV/AIDS organizations, indicated that the

---

[41]The AEA Roadmap states that evaluators should be professionals drawn from an interdisciplinary field that encompasses many areas of expertise, and with the appropriate training and experience for the evaluation activity.

evaluation team was employed by the program activity's implementing partner, but the report did not address potential conflict of interest.

Furthermore, some country and regional program evaluations sometimes did not provide enough identifying information about evaluators to allow an assessment of evaluator independence or qualifications. We estimate that 86 percent of the evaluations fully identified the evaluators, while 14 percent provided either partial or no information. For example, an evaluation report we reviewed relating to HIV prevention program activities in one region named the organization that conducted the evaluation but did not provide any information on the evaluation team members. Moreover, we were unable to find any information about this organization in an online search based on the limited information available in the report.

PEPFAR Evaluations Are Not All Publicly Disseminated

Agency policies and procedures generally support dissemination of evaluation results, but OGAC, CDC, and USAID have not ensured that evaluation methods, data, and evaluation results are made fully and easily accessible to the public.[42]

- **State.** State's newly released evaluation policy requires bureaus to submit evaluations to a central repository.

- **OGAC.** OGAC officials told us that the office supports dissemination of the results of important global HIV/AIDS research and evaluations to a variety of stakeholders. For example, OGAC officials noted that the PEPFAR website contains information on PEPFAR results as well as monitoring and evaluation guides. OGAC officials also noted that dissemination strategies are a common component of evaluation protocols and the procurement mechanisms that fund them. In addition, OGAC maintains an intranet site, which is accessible to PEPFAR implementing agency officials and contains information

---

[42]The AEA Roadmap states that federal agencies should publicly disseminate evaluation results systematically, broadly, and in a timely manner, making them easily accessible and usable through the Internet, and should make evaluation data and methods available to ensure transparency.

about evaluation. However, OGAC does not have a mechanism for publicly and systematically disseminating evaluation results.[43]

- **CDC.** CDC policy advises that effort is needed to ensure that evaluation findings are disseminated appropriately but does not require online dissemination of evaluation reports.[44] CDC officials told us that they recently made changes to CDC's public website, which, as of April 2012, includes some information on program evaluations. In addition, CDC's Division of Global HIV/AIDS (DGHA) Science Office maintains a catalog of published journal articles coauthored by DGHA officials. However, CDC does not maintain a complete online inventory of evaluations.

- **USAID.** USAID's policy states that evaluation findings should be shared as widely as possible with a commitment to full and active disclosure. USAID requires submission of completed evaluations to the Development Experience Clearinghouse (DEC), the agency's online repository of research documentation,[45] but does not enforce this requirement. In 2010, USAID reported that practices for disseminating evaluation results were generally limited, that dissemination practices varied across the agency, and that the requirement to submit completed evaluations to the DEC had not been fully enforced. Additionally, USAID found that documents in the DEC were sometimes difficult to find.[46] In February 2012, USAID also

---

[43]The Institute of Medicine recommended in 2007 that the U.S. Global AIDS Initiative increase its contribution to the global evidence base for HIV/AIDS programs by learning about and sharing what works. See Institute of Medicine, *PEPFAR Implementation: Progress and Promise* (Washington, D.C.: 2007).

[44]CDC's DGHA requires approval for public dissemination of reports and articles.

[45]The USAID evaluation policy requires each program office to submit both final evaluation results and summaries of its findings to the DEC within 3 months of their completion. This applies to both completed evaluation reports and the final drafts of any report submitted to USAID. The policy further requires evaluation data to be warehoused for future use but does not denote a specific repository for that purpose.

[46]The report also notes that USAID was designing the DEC to make it more user friendly and useful for USAID staff and external stakeholders. See USAID, *Report to Congress on Program Review and Evaluation Process* (Washington, D.C.: Mar. 30, 2011).

found that missions had reported submitting only 20 percent of their evaluations to the DEC in fiscal year 2009.[47]

Although documents submitted by 31 PEPFAR country and 3 regional teams showed that CDC and USAID have disseminated evaluation findings within these countries and regions in several ways, we found no publicly accessible and easily searchable Internet source for PEPFAR program evaluations. We received abstracts from annual meetings and conferences, presentations to partner government officials and stakeholders, published journal articles, and periodic agency reports, which may be publicly accessible via the Internet.[48] However, as of the time of our review, our searches of five key websites generated far fewer PEPFAR evaluations than the 496 evaluations we received from country teams, CDC and USAID headquarters, and OGAC.[49] We searched PubMed, the U.S. National Library of Medicine's online database, but a search using "PEPFAR" and "evaluation" as search terms generated seven results. Likewise, as of April 2012, our search of USAID's DEC, using "HIV/AIDS" and "evaluation" as search terms, generated 87 results, including some that were not evaluations, but USAID officials, in response to our request, later provided us nearly 300 evaluations. We also found some evaluations at two USAID-maintained websites, OVCsupport.net and AIDStar-One, but neither site was comprehensive or fully searchable.[50] In addition, a website called Global HIV M&E Information

---

[47]USAID also reported that, from 2010 to 2011, the agency had increased the number of evaluation reports submitted to the DEC. See USAID, *Evaluation Policy: Year One, First Annual Report and Plan for 2012 and 2013*.

[48]For example, country and regional teams submitted evaluations published in journals such as *The Lancet, Journal of Acquired Immune Deficiency Syndromes*, and *Journal of the American Medical Association*. In addition, CDC publishes evaluation research findings in its *Morbidity and Mortality Weekly Report*, CDC's "primary vehicle for scientific publication of timely, reliable, authoritative, accurate, objective, and useful public health information and recommendations." For more information, see www.cdc.gov/mmwr.

[49]According to CDC and OGAC officials, public dissemination may be limited by concerns raised by partner country ministries of health or implementing partners' copyright concerns.

[50]OVCsupport.net is an online repository for sharing information on programs supporting orphans and vulnerable children. For more information, see www.ovcsupport.net. AIDStar-One is managed by USAID's Implementation Support Division and provides "targeted assistance in knowledge management, program implementation support, technical leadership, program sustainability, and strategic planning." For more information, see www.aidstar-one.com.

provides a repository of voluntarily submitted monitoring and evaluation resources; however, we found few evaluations of PEPFAR programs.

Conclusions

PEPFAR's authorizing legislation emphasizes the importance of program evaluation as a tool for OGAC to ensure, among other things, that funds are spent on programs that show evidence of success. State, CDC, and USAID have demonstrated a clear commitment to program evaluation by conducting a wide variety of program evaluations that address at least one activity in each PEPFAR program area. However, many evaluations managed by PEPFAR country and regional teams lack fully supported findings, conclusions, and recommendations, evidenced by a lack of general adherence to common evaluation standards. Without fully supported findings, conclusions, and recommendations, these PEPFAR program evaluations have limited usefulness as a basis for decision making and may supply incomplete or misleading information for managers' and stakeholders' efforts to direct PEPFAR funding to programs that produce the desired outcomes and impacts.

State, CDC, and USAID have demonstrated their commitment to program evaluation by developing policies and procedures that apply to evaluations, in accordance with established general principles. However, without a requirement that country and regional teams prepare and submit annual evaluation plans—for example, as a component of operational plans—OGAC is unable to ensure that program activities are subject to appropriate levels of evaluation. Moreover, without documentation of the independence and competence of PEPFAR program evaluators, OGAC, agency program managers, and other stakeholders have limited assurance that evaluation results are unbiased and credible. Finally, unless evaluation results are publicly and systematically disseminated and made easily searchable online, program officials and public health researchers may be unable to assess the credibility of their findings or use them for program decision making.

Recommendations for Executive Action

We recommend that the Secretary of State direct the U.S. Global AIDS Coordinator to take the following four actions in collaboration with CDC and USAID to enhance PEPFAR evaluations:

1. develop a strategy to improve PEPFAR implementing agencies' and country and regional teams' adherence to common evaluation standards;

2. require implementing agency headquarters and country and regional teams to include evaluation plans in their annual operational plans;

3. provide detailed guidance for implementing agencies and country and regional teams on assessing, ensuring, and documenting the independence and competence of PEPFAR program evaluators; and

4. increase the online accessibility of PEPFAR program evaluation results.

Agency Comments

We provided a draft of this report to State, HHS's CDC, and USAID. Responding jointly with CDC and USAID, State OGAC provided written comments (see app. IV). CDC and USAID also provided technical comments, which we incorporated as appropriate.

In its written comments, State agreed with our recommendations and, emphasizing the interagency nature of the PEPFAR program, indicated that it will coordinate with PEPFAR agencies to implement our recommendations. First, State explained that it will work with PEPFAR implementing agencies to carry out the agencies' evaluation policies and practices, which State deemed generally consistent with AEA principles, and will develop strategies to ensure the appropriate application of common evaluation standards. Second, State responded that it will work through PEPFAR interagency processes to develop PEPFAR program evaluation plans, which it noted could be included in annual PEPFAR operational plans. Third, State will work with PEPFAR implementing agencies to put in place guidance to document program evaluators' independence and qualifications. Fourth, State affirmed that OGAC will collaborate with PEPFAR implementing agencies to develop strategies for improving dissemination of evaluation results and will use PEPFAR's public website to link to agencies' online resources.

We are sending copies of this report to the Secretary of State, the Office of the U.S. Global AIDS Coordinator, U.S. Agency for International Development's Office of HIV/AIDS, the Department of Health and Human Services' Office of Global Affairs, the Centers for Disease Control and Prevention's Division of Global HIV/AIDS, and appropriate congressional committees. In addition, the report is available at no charge on the GAO website at http://www.gao.gov.

If you or your staffs have any questions about this report, please contact me at (202) 512-3149 or gootnickd@gao.gov. Contact points for our Offices of Congressional Relations and Public Affairs may be found on the last page of this report. GAO staff who made major contributions to this report are listed in appendix VI.

David Gootnick
Director
International Affairs and Trade

The Honorable John Kerry
Chairman
The Honorable Richard G. Lugar
Ranking Member
Committee on Foreign Relations
United States Senate

The Honorable Patrick Leahy
Chairman
The Honorable Lindsey Graham
Ranking Member
Subcommittee on State, Foreign Operations,
   and Related Programs
Committee on Appropriations
United States Senate

The Honorable Ileana Ros-Lehtinen
Chairman
The Honorable Howard L. Berman
Ranking Member
Committee on Foreign Affairs
House of Representatives

The Honorable Kay Granger
Chairwoman
The Honorable Nita M. Lowey
Ranking Member
Subcommittee on State, Foreign Operations,
   and Related Programs
Committee on Appropriations
House of Representatives

Appendix I: Objectives, Scope, and Methodology

This report (1) identifies President's Emergency Plan for AIDS Relief (PEPFAR) evaluation activities and examines the extent to which evaluation results are supported and (2) examines the extent to which PEPFAR policies and procedures adhere to established principles for the evaluation of U.S. government programs. To identify PEPFAR program evaluations and examine the extent to which they generated supported evaluation results, we collected and analyzed program evaluation documents provided by Centers for Disease Control and Prevention (CDC) and U.S. Agency for International Development (USAID) officials in the 31 PEPFAR countries and 3 regions with PEPFAR country or regional operational plans in fiscal year 2010, as well as the Department of State's (State) Office of the U.S. Global AIDS Coordinator (OGAC) and CDC and USAID headquarters officials. To examine the extent to which PEPFAR program evaluation policies and procedures adhered to principles in the American Evaluation Association's (AEA) *An Evaluation Roadmap for a More Effective Government* (AEA Roadmap), we reviewed the general principles for conducting federal government program evaluations, as well as OGAC, State, USAID, and CDC policies and guidance. In addition, we surveyed CDC and USAID officials in the 31 PEPFAR countries and 3 regions with PEPFAR annual country or regional operational plans in fiscal year 2010, as well as CDC and USAID headquarters officials, regarding ongoing and completed evaluations. Finally, we conducted interviews with OGAC, CDC, and USAID officials in Washington, D.C., and Atlanta, Georgia.

Survey of PEPFAR Officials

To survey PEPFAR country and regional team officials, we took the following steps:

1. We consulted with OGAC and CDC and USAID headquarters officials and decided to use implementing mechanism[1] as a proxy for a program activity. We determined that using implementing mechanisms was the only viable unit of analysis to estimate the percentage of PEPFAR programs with evaluations because (1) OGAC officials maintained updated data on implementing mechanisms and (2) PEPFAR officials regularly used and understood data on implementing mechanisms. However, in some of these cases, if the

---

[1]An implementing mechanism is a grant, cooperative agreement, or contract in which a discrete dollar amount is passed through a prime implementing partner entity and for which the prime implementing partner is held fiscally accountable.

broader program was evaluated, not all implementing mechanisms under the larger program were necessarily evaluated. We also recognized that evaluations may not be appropriate for all implementing mechanisms (such as those that provide funding for staffing costs). To the extent possible, we eliminated these implementing mechanisms from our analysis.

2. We obtained lists of program activities for fiscal years 2008 through 2010 from OGAC for each country and region. We then analyzed program activities by country (or region) and agency; the lists included identification numbers, names, and partner names for each of the program activities. Each survey tool then contained a list of program activities relevant to the country or regional team.

3. Based on GAO and OGAC guidance, we developed the following working definition of evaluation: Evaluations are systematic studies to assess how well a program is working. Evaluations are often conducted by experts external to the program, either inside or outside the agency. Types of evaluations include process, outcome, impact, or cost-benefit analysis.

4. We developed a survey tool for ongoing and completed evaluations of PEPFAR programs. We consulted with OGAC and CDC and USAID headquarters officials about the survey tool and made revisions as appropriate. For example, based on input from CDC and USAID headquarters officials, we determined that some PEPFAR evaluations could address several implementing mechanisms. In addition, in some of these cases, if a broader program (e.g., national treatment program) was evaluated, not all implementing mechanisms under the broader program were necessarily evaluated. In response, we included questions in our survey prompting PEPFAR officials to indicate whether an implementing mechanism has been evaluated as part of a broader evaluation of several implementing mechanisms.

5. We tested the survey tool with officials in two PEPFAR countries—Angola and Ethiopia—and finalized the survey tool based on discussions with these officials.

6. We sent the final survey tool to PEPFAR country contacts (PEPFAR coordinators and CDC and USAID officials) identified by OGAC and CDC and USAID headquarters. The survey tool instructed CDC and USAID country or regional team officials to provide "yes" or "no"

responses to the following questions for each implementing
mechanism in the country's (or region's) agency-specific lists:

- Is this one of your agency's fiscal year 2008-2010 country or regional
operational plan program activities?

- Has at least one evaluation specific to this implementing mechanism
been completed?

- Is at least one evaluation specific to this implementing mechanism
ongoing?

- Has at least one evaluation covering, but broader than, this
implementing mechanism been completed?

- Is at least one evaluation covering, but broader than, this
implementing mechanism ongoing?

We also prompted the country or regional officials to provide additional
information for each implementing mechanism, such as explanations for
program activities that do not belong to the agency and identification of
duplicate program activities. Officials were instructed to either e-mail the
completed surveys to GAO or upload them to a website regularly used by
OGAC and country and regional teams for submitting and sharing
planning and reporting documents.

In some cases, we met with country or regional team officials via
telephone, or corresponded via e-mail, to clarify the purpose of the
survey, the questions themselves, and the evaluation document request
as well as to correct anomalies and ask follow-up questions. One GAO
analyst also attended the May 2011 PEPFAR implementing agency
annual meeting in Johannesburg, South Africa, to provide information
about the survey and evaluation document request to PEPFAR country
and regional team officials also attending the annual meeting. We
received responses from all 31 PEPFAR countries and 3 regions with
fiscal year 2010 operational plans.

Using a similar survey tool, we also conducted surveys of CDC and
USAID headquarters officials regarding program activities managed by
agency headquarters and listed in PEPFAR headquarters operational
plans for 2008 through 2010.

Analysis of Survey Responses

To analyze country and regional teams' survey responses, we made the following assumptions regarding the survey responses:

- If officials did not provide a response to the question "Is this one of your agency's fiscal year 2008-2010 country or regional operational plans program activities?" we included that implementing mechanism in the analysis. Program activities with responses of "no" or "duplicate" were eliminated from the analysis.

- If officials did not respond to any of the four questions regarding ongoing or completed evaluations, we assumed that there were no ongoing or completed evaluations for that implementing mechanism.

In addition, we reviewed narrative comments provided by country and regional team officials. We recognized that evaluations may not be appropriate for all implementing mechanisms (such as those that provide funding for staffing costs). To the extent possible, we eliminated these implementing mechanisms from our analysis. Based in part on our review of the narrative comments, we flagged and eliminated implementing mechanisms with evidence indicating that the implementing mechanism was either "to be determined" (i.e., the agency had yet to make an award to an implementing partner), related to staffing costs, related to strategic information and monitoring and evaluation, recently begun, a duplicate of another implementing mechanism, or listed in error.

Once the survey responses were ready for analysis, we calculated the summary statistics that are reported in the body of the report. We also included the survey responses provided by officials in CDC and USAID headquarters in the analysis. To check the reliability of the data analysis, a second independent analyst reviewed the statistical programs used to analyze the data for accuracy.

Program Evaluation Document Collection

In addition to our survey of CDC and USAID officials in the 31 countries and 3 regions with fiscal year 2011 operational plans, we requested program evaluation documents. To do this, the survey tool instructions prompted CDC and USAID officials to provide documentation of completed and ongoing evaluations. Specifically, for implementing mechanisms where officials indicated that at least one evaluation had been completed, we requested documentation—such as an evaluation report—of all such completed evaluations. For implementing mechanisms where officials indicated that at least one evaluation was ongoing, we requested documentation—such as terms of work or an evaluation plan.

We generally advised country and regional team officials to err on the
side of inclusion when in doubt about whether to submit documentation of
ongoing and completed evaluations. We instructed these officials to e-
mail, or, in some cases, mail electronic versions of the program
evaluation documents to GAO, or to upload them to a website regularly
used by OGAC and country and regional teams for submitting and
sharing planning and reporting documents.

In response to this document request, we received more than 1,350
documents. For example, we received documentation of ongoing or
planned evaluations, such as statements of work or evaluation protocols
and protocol approval forms. We also received meeting minutes, trip
reports, financial review and audit documents, presentation slides,
abstracts, and conference posters. To determine which documents met
our definition of evaluation, we reviewed each of these documents and
categorized them as meeting the definition of evaluation or not, following
a set of decision rules. For example, we included data quality
assessments, costing studies that compared costs and explained cost
differences, and analyses of surveillance data pre- and postintervention.
We excluded surveillance studies that simply reported the results of a
surveillance activity (but did not link it to a specific program or
intervention); needs assessments, baseline studies, and situation
analyses; trip and site visit reports; and pre- and postevent (e.g.,
workshop) questionnaires or surveys. We identified and eliminated
duplicate documents. This categorization was checked by a second
analyst and yielded 436 program evaluations. We believe that this final
set of evaluations constitutes an essentially full universe of PEPFAR
country and regional program evaluation documents.

In addition to the program evaluation documents collected from CDC and
USAID officials in PEPFAR countries and regions, we requested
documents from OGAC related to PEPFAR public health evaluations. We
also requested evaluation documents related to PEPFAR program
managed by CDC and USAID headquarters from officials at each
agency's headquarters. OGAC provided copies of 18 completed public
health evaluations, CDC headquarters provided copies of 22 completed
evaluations, and USAID headquarters provided copies of 24 completed
evaluations.

We reviewed the program evaluation documents submitted by PEPFAR
country and regional teams as well as CDC and USAID headquarters
officials. We identified whether each program evaluation was ongoing or
completed as well as which program area or areas (e.g., prevention,

treatment, care, or other) were evaluated. To do this, we used program categories defined by OGAC's fiscal years 2011 operational plan guidance, resulting in the program areas and related areas reported in the report. This categorization was checked by a second analyst. Table 4 provided descriptions of the PEPFAR program areas.

Table 4: PEPFAR Program Area Descriptions

Program area	Description
Prevention	
Prevention of mother-to-child transmission (PMTCT)	Activities aimed at preventing mother-to-child HIV transmission, including antiretroviral prophylaxis for HIV-infected pregnant women and newborns and counseling and support for maternal nutrition.
Abstinence/be faithful	Activities to promote abstinence, including delay of sexual activity or secondary abstinence, fidelity, reducing multiple and concurrent partners, and related social and community norms that impact these behaviors. Activities address programming for both adolescents and adults.
Other sexual prevention	Activities aimed at preventing HIV transmission, including purchase and promotion of condoms, management of sexually transmitted infections, and programs to reduce other risks of persons engaged in high-risk behaviors. Prevention services should be focused on target populations such as alcohol users; at risk youth; men who have sex with men; mobile populations, including migrant workers, truck drivers, and members of military and other uniformed services; and persons who exchange sex for money, other goods, or both with multiple or concurrent sex partners, including persons engaged in prostitution, transactional sexual partnerships, or both.
Blood safety	Activities supporting a nationally coordinated blood program to ensure a safe and adequate blood supply, including infrastructure and policies; donor-recruitment activities; blood collection, testing for transfusion-transmissible infections, component preparation, storage, and distribution; appropriate clinical use of blood, transfusion procedures, and hemovigilance; training and human resource development; monitoring and evaluation; and development of sustainable systems.
Injection safety	Policies, training, waste-management systems, advocacy, and other activities to promote medical injection safety, including distribution/supply chain, cost and appropriate disposal of injection equipment, and other related equipment and supplies.
Medical male circumcision (MC)	Policy, training, outreach, message development, service delivery, quality assurance, and equipment and commodities related to male circumcision. All MC services should include the minimum package; HIV testing and counseling provided on-site; age-appropriate pre- and postoperative sexual risk reduction counseling; active exclusion of symptomatic sexually transmitted infections and syndromic treatment when indicated; provision and promotion of correct and consistent use of condoms; circumcision surgery in accordance with national standards and international guidance; counseling on the need for abstinence from sexual activity during wound healing; wound care instructions; and postoperative clinical assessments and care.
Prevention among injecting and noninjecting drug users	Activities including policy reform, training, message development, community mobilization, and comprehensive approaches, including medication assistance therapy to reduce injecting drug use. Procurement of methadone and other medical-assisted therapy drugs should be included under this program area budget code. Programs for prevention of sexual transmission within injecting drug users should be included in this category.
Counseling and testing	Activities in which both HIV counseling and testing are provided for those who seek to know their HIV status or provider-initiated testing and counseling.

Program area	Description
Care	
Adult care and support	All facility-based and home/community-based activities for HIV-infected adults and their families aimed at extending and optimizing quality of life for HIV-infected clients and their families throughout the continuum of illness through provision of clinical, psychological, spiritual, social, and prevention services. Clinical care should include prevention and treatment of opportunistic infections (excluding TB) and other HIV/AIDS-related complications, including malaria and diarrhea (providing access to commodities such as pharmaceuticals, insecticide-treated nets, safe water interventions, and related laboratory services); pain and symptom relief; and nutritional assessment and support, including food. Psychological and spiritual support may include group and individual counseling and culturally appropriate end-of-life care and bereavement services. Social support may include vocational training, income-generating activities, social and legal protection, and training and support of caregivers. Prevention services may include "prevention for positives" behavioral counseling and counseling and testing of family members.
Pediatric care and support	All health facility-based care for HIV-exposed children aimed at extending and optimizing quality of life for HIV-infected clients and their families throughout the continuum of illness through provision of clinical, psychological, spiritual, social, and prevention services. Clinical care should include early infant diagnosis, prevention and treatment of opportunistic infections (excluding TB) and other HIV/AIDS-related complications, including malaria and diarrhea (providing access to commodities such as pharmaceuticals, insecticide treated nets, safe water interventions, and related laboratory services); pain and symptom relief; and nutritional assessment and support, including targeted food interventions. Other services, such as psychological, social, spiritual, and prevention services, should be provided as appropriate.
Orphans and vulnerable children (OVC)	Activities aimed at improving the lives of orphans and other vulnerable children affected by HIV/AIDS, and doing so in a measurable way. Services to children (0-17 years) should be based on the actual needs of each child and could include ensuring access to basic education (from early childhood development through secondary level); basic health care services; targeted food and nutrition support, including support for safe infant feeding and weaning practices; protection; mitigation of factors that place children at risk; legal aid; economic strengthening; training of caregivers in HIV prevention and home-based care; and so forth. Household-centered approaches that link OVC services with HIV-affected families (linkages with PMTCT, palliative care, treatment, etc.) and strengthen the capacity of the family unit (caregiver) are included along with strengthening community structures that protect and promote healthy child development (schools, churches, clinics, child protection committees, etc.) and investments in local and national government capacity to identify, monitor, and track children's well-being. Programs may be included that strengthen the transition from residential OVC care to more family-centered models.
TB/HIV	Exams, clinical monitoring, related laboratory services, treatment, and prevention of tuberculosis (including medications); HIV testing and clinical care of clients in TB service locations; TB screening; and diagnosis, treatment and prevention of TB in people living with HIV/AIDS. Funding for these activities, including commodities and laboratory, should be included in the TB/HIV budget code rather than other budget codes. The location of TB/HIV activities can include general medical settings, HIV/AIDS clinics, home-based care, and traditional TB clinics and hospitals.
Treatment	
Antiretroviral (ARV) drugs	Procurement, delivery, and transport of ARV drugs, including all antiretroviral postexposure prophylaxis procurement for rape victims.
Adult treatment	Infrastructure, training clinicians and other providers, exams, clinical monitoring, related laboratory services, and community-adherence activities.
Pediatric treatment	Infrastructure, training clinicians and other providers, exams, clinical monitoring, related laboratory services, and community-adherence activities.
Other	
Laboratory infrastructure	Development and strengthening of laboratory systems and facilities to support HIV/AIDS-related activities, including purchase of equipment and commodities and provision of quality assurance, staff training, and other technical assistance.

Program area	Description
Strategic information	HIV/AIDS behavioral and biological surveillance; facility surveys; monitoring of partner results; reporting of results; support of health information systems; assistance to countries in establishing such systems, strengthening them, or both; and related analyses and data dissemination activities.
Health systems strengthening	Activities that contribute to national-, regional-, or district-level health systems by supporting finance, leadership and governance (including broad policy reform efforts, including addressing stigma, gender issues, etc.), human resources for health, institutional capacity building, supply chain or procurement systems, information systems, Global Fund programs, and donor coordination.

Source: GAO synthesis of OGAC information provided in fiscal year 2012 country and regional operational plan guidance.

Development of Evaluation Assessment Tool

To determine the degree to which these evaluations were conducted in adherence with common evaluation standards, we used an assessment tool to systematically conduct in-depth analyses of a probability sample of the evaluations submitted by the PEPFAR country and regional teams and a nonprobability sample of the evaluations submitted by OGAC and CDC and USAID headquarters officials. Our PEPFAR evaluation assessment tool was based on an assessment tool used for a prior GAO report, which we updated using guidance on evaluation from USAID,[2] CDC,[3] the Organization for Economic Cooperation and Development (OECD),[4] and GAO. We piloted the assessment tool with three PEPFAR program evaluation documents provided by CDC and USAID headquarters officials and revised the evaluation assessment as appropriate. After piloting and revising the tool, we finalized the tool and used it to conduct the in-depth analyses of program evaluation documents. Table 5 lists the questions and supporting questions included in the assessment tool.

[2]We used USAID's 2010 guidance, which was in effect for fiscal years 2008 through 2010 (the time frame used to request evaluations from implementing agency headquarters and country and regional team officials).

[3]See Department of Health and Human Services, Centers for Disease Control and Prevention, "Framework for Program Evaluation in Public Health" *Morbidity and Mortality Weekly Report: Recommendations and Reports*, vol. 48, no. RR-11 (1999), accessed October 2011, http://www.cdc.gov/eval/framework/index.htm.

[4]See OECD, Development Assistance Committee Guidelines and Reference Series, *Quality Standards for Development Evaluation* (Paris: April 2010), available at http://www.oecd.org/dataoecd/55/0/44798177.pdf.

Table 5: Questions Included in the GAO Evaluation Assessment Tool

Assessment questions	Supporting questions
Does the evaluation specify why the evaluation is needed?	• Is the hypothesis or rationale underlying the program identified? • Are any related evaluations, studies, or other documents (e.g., mid-term evaluation) identified?
Does the evaluation identify stakeholders?	
Does the evaluation identify program and evaluation objectives?	• Are the program or intervention objectives identified? • Are the evaluation objectives identified? • Is the reason (i.e., intended use or purpose) for deciding to conduct an evaluation identified? • Is the link between program and evaluation objectives identified? • Is any information provided on how evaluation results should be used for decision making?
Does the evaluation identify evaluation criteria?	• Have the criteria or standards that will be used to measure performance been identified?
Does the evaluation identify the evaluation team and any conflicts of interest?	• Is the evaluation team composition identified? • Are potential conflicts of interest identified and/or addressed?
Does the evaluation identify time frames for conducting the evaluation?	
Does the evaluation design appear to be appropriate?	• Is the overall evaluation design identified? • Have the assumptions underlying the design been articulated? • Have design limitations been identified? If so, are the ways in which these limitations were addressed identified? • Overall, is the identified evaluation design appropriate to answer the evaluation questions?

Do participant/sample selection methods and sample size appear to be generally appropriate?	• What are the criteria for selecting or sampling participants, respondents, or other entities?
	• Is participant selection bias acknowledged? If so, was it addressed?
	• If probability sampling is used:
	  • Is the sampling strategy appropriate?
	  • Is the sampling frame appropriate?
	  • Is the sampling unit described?
	• If nonprobability sampling is used, is the sampling strategy appropriate?
	• If this is a comparison study, does it address how participants, respondents, or other units are assigned to the comparison groups or selected more generally?
	• If the evaluation involves human subjects, have Institutional Review Board or other human subjects review approval procedures been identified?
	• Have sample size calculations (e.g., confidence intervals) or limitations been identified?

Assessment questions	Supporting questions
Do the measures used for this evaluation appear to be appropriate?	• Have the key measures—that is, input, output, outcome, and/or impact—been identified?
	• Are measures clearly linked to evaluation questions?
	• Do the identified measures appear to be appropriate for answering the evaluation questions?
	• For pre-, post-, or comparison group evaluations, is there parallel measurement for comparison groups—that is, were the same data collected for comparison and treatment groups?
	• Have possible confounding effects been identified, measured, and/or controlled for?
	• If an instrument (e.g., survey or data collection instrument) is used to measure key variables, does it appear to be reliable and valid?
	• Has the possibility of negative side effects or unintended outcomes been considered?
	• If appropriate, are alternative explanations of the measured impacts discussed?
Do the data collection and analysis methods appear to be appropriate?	• Are data collection methods and procedures discussed?
	• Are data analysis methods and procedures discussed?
	• Are data collection and/or database management controls identified?
	• Were any robustness checks on the methodology or sensitivity analysis conducted?
	• Are issues related to nonrespondents, dropouts, or missing data identified and/or addressed?
Are the evaluation results specified?	• Are the following clearly documented?
	• Evaluation findings/results
	• Conclusions
	• Recommendations
	• Lessons learned
	• Stakeholder comments
	• What are the key evaluation findings/results?
	• What are the key evaluation conclusions?
	• What are the recommendations?
Based on the analysis of the elements above, do the evaluation findings/results, conclusions, and recommendations appear to be supported?	

Source: GAO.

Sampling from Program Evaluation Documents Submitted by PEPFAR Country and Regional Teams

To allow us to generalize to the entire set of evaluations provided by PEPFAR country and regional teams, we randomly selected a sample of 84 of 436 evaluations submitted by CDC and USAID officials in 31 PEPFAR countries and 3 regions. The list of all evaluations was sorted by total approved operational plan budgets for each country or region for fiscal years 2008 through 2010, so that a systematic sample would ensure representation of countries with relatively large, medium, and small budgets for fiscal years 2008 through 2011.

After sampling, 6 evaluations—including, for example, baseline and feasibility studies—were found to be out of scope, resulting in a final

sample of 78. Results based on random probability samples are subject
to sampling error. The sample we drew for our survey is only one of a
large number of samples we might have drawn. Because different
samples could have provided different estimates, we express our
confidence in the precision of our particular sample results as a 95
percent confidence interval. This is the interval that would contain the
actual population values for 95 percent of the samples we could have
drawn. The margin of error associated with proportion estimates is no
more than plus or minus 11 percentage points at the 95 percent level of
confidence and estimates of totals have a margin of error no larger than
44 evaluations.

For the 18 public health evaluations submitted by OGAC, as well as the
20 and 22 evaluations submitted by CDC and USAID headquarters,
respectively, we selected a nonprobability sample based on the type of
program (e.g., prevention, treatment, care, or other) evaluated as well as
country or countries addressed by each evaluation. Because this is a
nonprobability sample, the results of our assessments of these
evaluations cannot be used to make inferences about all evaluations
managed by OGAC and CDC and USAID headquarters. However, they
do represent a mix of the types of evaluations managed by OGAC and
CDC and USAID headquarters.

Assessing Program Evaluation Documents

Using our evaluation assessment tool, we conducted in-depth analyses of
the evaluation documents submitted by the PEPFAR country and regional
teams and also those submitted by OGAC, USAID, and CDC
headquarters. To do so, one analyst conducted an initial review of the
evaluation document and then completed the evaluation assessment tool.
The analyst also recorded basic information about each evaluation,
including title, author, date of publication, and the country or countries
included in the evaluation. For each of the questions in the assessment
tool (see table 1), analysts were instructed to (1) respond using "yes,"
"no," "partial," "not sure," or "not applicable" and (2) summarize or cite
relevant information from the evaluation documents. Analysts then were
instructed to weigh the evidence and answers to these questions and
provide "yes," "no," "partial,", "not sure," or "not applicable" responses for
each category. Based on the analysis of the elements addressed in the
assessment tool, analysts determined the extent to which each
evaluation's findings, conclusions, and recommendations were supported
using "yes," "no," "partial," or "not sure" as their responses. This overall
determination was not based on a tally of responses to individual
elements in the evaluation assessment tool, but rather a synthesis of

these responses and an assessment of the contribution of each element to the overall support for the evaluation's findings, conclusions, and recommendations. To help ensure consistency in the application of the standards and questions, the assessors met weekly during the assessment period to clarify the instructions and discuss their observations. After each assessment was complete, a second analyst independently verified the results of the analysis by reviewing the program evaluation document and the completed evaluation assessment tool. In cases where the two analysts did not concur on the results, or where there was a "not sure" response, they met to discuss the evidence and documented a final determination. All the results for the evaluation assessment tools were then entered into a spreadsheet and analyzed.

Analyzing Data Generated by Evaluation Assessments

To assess potential associations between key attributes of the sample of 78 evaluations we randomly selected, we calculated chi-square tests and the associated odds ratios for all pairs of the following variables: agency, methods used, evaluation type, and program type. Key results from these analyses are presented in the report. Additional results can be found in appendix III. We also employed logistic regressions to assess which of these variables (i.e., agency, methods used, evaluation type, and program type) had the strongest effects on the extent to which sampled evaluations contained support for findings, conclusions, and recommendations.

Assessing State, OGAC, CDC, and USAID Evaluation Policies

To assess State, OGAC, CDC, and USAID evaluation policies, we developed an assessment tool based on nine AEA Roadmap principles.[5] For each principle, we developed a question or series of questions asking how the policies addressed the AEA Roadmap principles. One analyst reviewed each agency's policy and filled out the tool by citing evidence that would support the policy's consistency with the AEA Roadmap principle, or a conclusion that no evidence could be found to support adherence to the principle. The analyst then concluded whether the policy was consistent with each principle assessed. A second analyst conducted a review of the completed assessment tools and either concurred with or disputed the conclusion for each principle. In cases where the two

---

[5]The AEA Roadmap principles include scope, coverage, analytic approaches and methods, resources, professional competence, evaluation plans, dissemination of evaluation results, evaluation policies and procedures, and independence.

analysts did not concur, they met to discuss the evidence and made a
final determination.

To determine the extent to which operational plans contained evaluation
plans, we reviewed OGAC's fiscal year 2011 and 2012 annual guidance
to implementing agency headquarters regarding development of the
annual PEPFAR headquarters operational plan. We documented
instances where the guidance addressed program evaluation and
determined whether it constituted instructions to develop an evaluation
plan. We conducted similar analysis of OGAC's fiscal year 2011 and 2012
annual guidance to PEPFAR country and regional teams to identify
instances where the guidance addressed evaluation and, finally, to
determine whether the guidance constituted instructions for developing
evaluation plans. In addition, we assessed 11 of the 33 country
operational plans and 2 of the 3 regional operational plans submitted to
OGAC for fiscal year 2011, the most recent year in which plans were
available. We documented instances where these operational plans
discussed evaluation and whether they contained evaluation plans.

To determine the extent to which the program evaluations documented
potential conflicts of interest and the identity of evaluators, we included
questions on these two elements in our evaluation assessment tool.
Analysts were instructed to respond using "yes," "no," or "partial" to these
questions and to cite relevant evidence. After each assessment was
complete, a second analyst verified the results of the analysis by
reviewing the program evaluation document and the completed
evaluation assessment tool. In cases where the two analysts did not
concur on the results, they met to discuss the evidence and documented
a final determination. All the results for the evaluation assessment tools
were then entered into a spreadsheet and analyzed.

We searched five Internet databases referenced by OGAC, CDC, and
USAID officials to determine the public accessibility of PEPFAR program
evaluations. These five sites included the Development Experience
Clearinghouse (http://dec.usaid.gov/index.cfm), PubMed
(http://www.ncbi.nlm.nih.gov/pubmed/), OVCsupport.net
(http://www.ovcsupport.net/s/), AIDSTAR-One (http://www.aidstar-
one.com/), and Global HIV M&E Info
(https://www.globalhivmeinfo.org/Pages/HomePage.aspx). For each of
these websites, we conducted searches using keywords that would
capture any PEPFAR-related program evaluations or documentation,
such as "PEPFAR," "evaluation," and "HIV/AIDS." Where applicable, we
then captured the results and counted the number of documents that

could reasonably be considered documentation of a PEPFAR program
evaluation.

We conducted this performance audit from August 2011 to May 2012 in
accordance with generally accepted government auditing standards.
Those standards require that we plan and perform the audit to obtain
sufficient, appropriate evidence to provide a reasonable basis for our
findings and conclusions based on our audit objectives. We believe that
the evidence obtained provides a reasonable basis for our findings and
conclusions based on our audit objectives.

Appendix II: GAO Evaluation Definitions and Standards

Past GAO work has emphasized evaluation as a key source of information to help agency officials and Congress make decisions about the programs they oversee.[1] GAO distinguishes performance measurement—the ongoing monitoring and reporting of program accomplishments—from evaluation, which is defined as individual, systematic studies conducted periodically or on an ad hoc basis to assess how well a program is working.[2] Further, according to GAO guidance, experts external to the program, program managers, or both conduct evaluations to examine the performance of a program within a given context to understand not only whether a program works but also how to improve results. GAO guidance identifies four types of evaluation:

- *Process evaluation.* This type of evaluation assesses the degree to which a program is operating as it was intended. It typically assesses program activities' conformance to statutory or regulatory requirements, program design, and professional standards or customer expectations.

- *Outcome evaluation.* This type of evaluation assesses the degree to which a program achieves its outcome-oriented objectives. It focuses on outputs and outcomes (including unintended effects) to judge program effectiveness, but may also assess program process to understand how outcomes are produced.

- *Impact evaluation.* This is a form of outcome evaluation that assesses the net effect of a program by comparing program outcomes with an estimate of what would have happened in the absence of the program. Impact evaluation is used when external factors are known to influence the program's outcomes, in order to isolate the program's contribution to achievement of its objectives.

- *Cost-benefit or cost-effectiveness analysis.* This type of evaluation compares a program's outputs or outcomes with the costs to produce them. Cost-effectiveness analysis assesses the cost of meeting a single objective and can be used to identify the least costly alternative for meeting that goal.

---

[1]See GAO, *Program Evaluation: Experienced Agencies Follow a Similar Model for Prioritizing Research*, GAO-11-176 (Washington, D.C.: Jan. 14, 2011).

[2]See GAO, *Performance Measurement and Evaluation: Definitions and Relationships*, GAO-11-646SP (Washington, D.C.: May 2011).

In addition, GAO guidance provides basic information about the more
commonly used evaluation methods; introduces key issues in planning
evaluation studies of federal programs to best meet decision makers'
needs; and describes different types of evaluations for answering varied
questions about program performance, the process of designing
evaluation studies, and key issues to consider in ensuring overall study
quality. Further, the guidance recommends standards for evaluation
design, including establishing evaluation objectives, identifying
constraints, and assessing the appropriateness of the evaluation design.[3]

[3]See GAO, *Designing Evaluations: 2012 Revision*, GAO-12-208G (Washington, D.C.:
January 2012).

Appendix III: Statistical Comparison of PEPFAR Evaluations

We conducted a statistical analysis of the adequacy of support for findings in evaluations provided to us by CDC and USAID, to determine whether the adequacy of support differed by agency, by methods used, or by type of evaluation. Our analysis indicated that fully supported findings were more likely in CDC's evaluations than in USAID's evaluations; in evaluations that used quantitative methods than in evaluations that used qualitative or mixed methods;[1] and in cost-benefit or impact evaluations, as well as outcome evaluations, than in process evaluations. However, while CDC's evaluations' findings were more likely to be fully supported than USAID's evaluations' findings, the difference was not statistically significant after we accounted for the method used in the evaluations. This lack of statistical significance suggests that the difference was driven partly by the agencies' choice of evaluation method.[2]

Table 6 shows technical details of our statistical analysis of the level of support for findings in CDC and USAID evaluations.

---

[1]Qualitative methods include collecting data through interviews, focus groups, document or literature reviews, and observation, and analyzing data by discerning, examining, comparing, and contrasting meaningful patterns or themes in qualitative data. Quantitative methods typically involve collecting quantifiable information through probability sampling and using various forms of statistical analysis to generalize results. Evaluations using mixed methods employ a combination of qualitative and quantitative data collection and analysis techniques.

[2]Additional analyses (not shown) indicate that 67 percent of the CDC evaluations and 15 percent of the USAID evaluations used quantitative methods.

Table 6: Statistical Analysis of Support for Findings in CDC and USAID Evaluations, by Agency, Methods Used, and Type of Evaluation

	Support for findings			Odds on full support	Odds ratios
	Partial or none	Full	Total		
Total	**46**	**32**	**78**		
	59.0%	41.0%	**100.0%**		
By agency					
CDC	12	18	**30**	1.50	3.64
	40.0%	60.0%	**100.0%**		
USAID	34	14	**48**	0.41	REF
	70.8%	29.2%	**100.0%**		
Chi-square statistic (L^2) = 7.28 with 1 degree of freedom, P-value = .007					
By methods used					
Qualitative or mixed	41	10	**51**	0.24	REF
	80.4%	19.6%	**100.0%**		
Quantitative	5	22	**27**	4.40	18.04
	18.5%	81.5%	**100.0%**		
Chi-square statistic (L^2) = 29.25 with 1 degree of freedom, P-value < .001					
By type of evaluation					
Cost-benefit or impact	2	10	**12**	5.00	23.00
	16.7%	83.3%	**100.0%**		
Outcome	21	17	**38**	0.81	3.72
	55.3%	44.7%	**100.0%**		
Process	23	5	**28**	0.22	REF
	82.1%	17.9%	**100.0%**		
Chi-square statistic (L^2) = 16.26 with 2 degrees of freedom, P-value < .001					

Source: GAO analysis of CDC and USA D evaluations.

Notes:

We collapsed two categories of the dependent variable, "support for findings," into one category, collapsing "partial support" and "no support" into "partial or none." We also collapsed categories of the two independent variables: for the variable "methods used," we collapsed "qualitative methods" and "mixed methods" into "qualitative or mixed methods," and for "type of evaluation," we collapsed "cost-benefit evaluations" and "impact evaluations" into "cost-benefit or impact." We collapsed these categories after preliminary investigations revealed that doing so would result in no statistically significant loss of information. These preliminary investigations involved comparing likelihood-ratio chi-square statistics for expanded and collapsed versions of the tables. Where the difference in chi-squares for the tables compared is not significant, given the difference in degrees of freedom, it can reasonably be concluded that no significant information was lost as a result of collapsing.

REF signifies the category chosen as the referent category, or denominator, in calculating the odds ratios.

In table 6, the chi-square statistics at the base of each of the three panels show that the adequacy of support for findings varied significantly between the two agencies and differed significantly based on the methods used and type of evaluations. The odds ratios in the far-right column show that the odds of evaluations' being fully supported were 3.6 times greater for CDC than for USAID; 18 times greater for quantitative evaluations than for qualitative or mixed-methods evaluations; 23 times greater for cost-benefit or impact evaluations than for process evaluations; and 3.7 times greater for outcome evaluations than for process evaluations.[3]

In addition, we estimated binary logistic regression models to determine whether the difference in adequacy of support for findings in CDC's and USAID's evaluations resulted from differences in the methods used or differences in the types of evaluations conducted.[4] Table 7 shows the odds ratios that result from fitting logistic regression models to estimate the effects of the three different factors (agency, methods used, and type of evaluation) on the adequacy of support for findings. Models 1, 2, and 3 are bivariate models, which regress "support" on dummy variables for agency, methods used, and type of evaluation, with each variable considered one at a time. These produce the same odds ratios that we obtained from the observed data in table 6. In contrast, model 4 estimates the effects of agency and methods simultaneously, and model 5 estimates the effects of agency and type of evaluation. In comparing these models, we found that controlling for the methods used (model 4) rendered insignificant the differences between agencies in adequacy of

---

[3]To calculate the odds on findings' being fully supported in CDC evaluations (shown in table 6 under "Odds on full support"), we divided the number of evaluations with full support by the number with partial or no support (18/12 = 1.5). We performed a similar calculation of odds on findings' being fully supported in USAID evaluations (14/34 = 0.41). The results of these calculations imply that 1.5 CDC evaluations were fully supported for every CDC evaluation that was not, while 0.41 USAID evaluations were fully supported for every evaluation that was not. The ratio of these two odds—1.50/0.41 = 3.64 (shown in the far-right column of table 6)—shows that the odds on evaluation findings' being fully supported were 3.6 times greater for CDC than for USAID.

[4]A June 2011 assessment of 56 USAID evaluations—including 8 evaluations of programs funded at least in part through PEPFAR—found that the majority of the evaluations used mixed methods and that about a fourth of the evaluations employed quasi-experimental or statistical evaluation methods. See Office of the Director of U.S. Foreign Assistance, *A Meta Evaluation of Foreign Assistance Evaluations* (Washington, D.C.: 2011), accessed March 2011, http://pdf.usaid.gov/pdf_docs/PCAAC273.pdf.

support for findings, whereas controlling for type of evaluation (model 5)
did not.

**Table 7: Odds Ratios from Logistic Regression Models, Where Support for Findings
Was Regressed on Agency, Methods Used, and Type of Evaluation**

	Model				
Effects included	**1**	**2**	**3**	**4**	**5**
CDC	3.64[a]			0.88	3.90[a]
Quantitative methods		18.04[a]		19.38[a]	
Cost-benefit or impact evaluation			23.00[a]		21.04[a]
Outcome evaluation			3.72[a]		4.94[a]

Source: GAO analysis of CDC and USA D evaluations.

Note: The three-category variable representing the type of evaluation requires two dummy variables,
one contrasting the cost-benefit or impact evaluation with the process evaluations, and the other
contrasting the outcome evaluations with process evaluations.

[a]Odds ratio is statistically significant at the .05 level.

Appendix IV: Comments from the Department of State

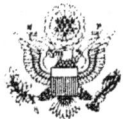

United States Department of State

Chief Financial Officer

Washington, D.C. 20520

Dr. Loren Yager
Managing Director
International Affairs and Trade
Government Accountability Office
441 G Street, N.W.
Washington, D.C. 20548-0001

MAY 2 1 2012

Dear Dr. Yager:

We appreciate the opportunity to review your draft report, "PRESIDENT EMERGENCY PLAN FOR AIDS RELIEF: Agencies Can Enhance Evaluation Quality, Planning, and Dissemination" GAO Job Code 320857.

The enclosed Department of State comments are provided for incorporation with this letter as an appendix to the final report.

If you have any questions concerning this response, please contact Leigh Ann Monk-Reyes, Program Support Officer, Office of the U.S. Global AIDS Coordinator at (202) 663-2753.

Sincerely,

James L. Millette

cc: GAO – David Gootnick
S/GAC– Eric Goosby
State/OIG – Evelyn Klemstine

Department of State Comments on GAO Draft Report

PRESIDENT'S EMERGENCY PLAN FOR AIDS RELIEF: Agencies Can Enhance Evaluation Quality, Planning, and Dissemination

(GAO-12-673, GAO Code 320857)

Thank you for the opportunity to comment on your draft report entitled, *"President's Emergency Plan For AIDS Relief: Agencies Can Enhance Evaluation Quality, Planning, and Dissemination, GAO-12-673, Job Code 320857."*

The GAO report included four recommendations for the Department of State's Office of the U.S. Global AIDS Coordinator (S/GAC).

The Department of States' Office of the U.S. Global AIDS Coordinator (S/GAC) and the PEPFAR implementing agencies appreciate the work conducted by the GAO to produce these findings and this draft report. These results reflect an earlier phase of the larger PEPFAR evaluation efforts, and although this work has improved, some of these findings remain equally valid today. This GAO report provides guidance on several issues, and S/GAC will coordinate with the implementing agencies to carry out these recommendations.

First, GAO recommends that the State Department coordinate with the Center for Disease Control (CDC) and United States Agency for International Development (USAID) to improve the PEPFAR implementing agencies' and country and regional teams' adherence to common evaluation standards. In response, State agrees to support the partner agencies in their implementation of agency evaluation policies and practices. These agency policies are generally consistent with the GAO-cited AEA standards. Headquarters based evaluations generally comply with these standards, but more effort will be important in each country. Different types of evaluations are conducted typically in the HQ (e.g., impact, outcome, operations research) and country (e.g., output, process, formative) settings, and S/GAC and PEPFAR partners will work over this next year to develop strategies to ensure the appropriate application of these standards accordingly.

Second, GAO recommends that State require its CDC and USAID implementing agency headquarters, and country and regional teams, to include PEPFAR evaluation plans in their respective annual operational plans. In response, State agrees and will work through interagency processes to define

2

overall PEPFAR evaluation objectives and plan, and apply this framework to
agency-specific plans to account for PEPFAR-supported work and to evaluation
planning for appropriate PEPFAR-supported countries. This latter effort requires
collaborative planning with National partner governments and stakeholders. An
evaluation plan also should be considered in conjunction with a broader research
agenda for each country. These processes demand considerable effort in-country,
and in the context of ongoing programmatic issues, this work will evolve over the
next couple of years. The annual operational plan can be used as a mechanism to
submit and update plans, once they have been developed.

Third, GAO recommends that State, CDC and USAID provide detailed
guidance at implementing agency headquarters and to country and regional teams
on assessing, ensuring, and documenting the independence and competence of
PEPFAR program evaluator qualifications. In response, State agrees and will
support agencies in the application of this standard to evaluation studies. Among
HQ supported studies, a peer-review process ensures compliance with these
recommendations. In-country studies typically are not as rigorous in design or
objective, but over the next year S/GAC will work with the implementing agencies
to develop and implement protocols to document the competence and appropriate
independence of evaluators.

Fourth, GAO recommends that State, CDC and USAID increase on-line
accessibility of PEPFAR evaluation results. In response, State agrees and will
collaborate with and support agency partners in the implementation of agency
dissemination practices. This work will involve assessing the current status of online dissemination activities and platforms, leading to development of agency
strategies to strengthen these efforts and improve the availability of evaluation
results. S/GAC also will develop the www.PEPFAR.gov website to maximize
linkages to these agency resources and expanding access to this information.

Appendix V: GAO Contact and Staff Acknowledgments

GAO Contact	David Gootnick, (202) 512-3149 or gootnickd@gao.gov
Staff Acknowledgments	In addition to the contact named above, Jim Michels, Assistant Director; Todd M. Anderson; Chad Davenport; David Dornisch; Lorraine Ettaro; Justin Fisher; Brian Hackney; Kay Halpern; Fang He; Reid Lowe; Grace Lui; and Erika Navarro made key contributions to this report. In addition to these staff, the following GAO staff assisted by conducting in-depth assessments of selected evaluations: Sada Aksartova, Gergana Danailova-Trainor, Leah DeWolf, Rachel Girshick, Jordan Holt, Kara Marshall, Jeff Miller, Steven Putansu, Mona Sehgal, and Doug Sloane. Sushmita Srikanth and Katy Crosby assisted with quality assurance reviews.

Related GAO Products

President's Emergency Plan for AIDS Relief: Program Planning and Reporting. GAO-11-785. Washington, D.C.: July 29, 2011.

Global Health: Trends in U.S. Spending for Global HIV/AIDS and Other Health Assistance in Fiscal Years 2001-2008. GAO-11-64. Washington, D.C.: October 8, 2010.

President's Emergency Plan for AIDS Relief: Efforts to Align Programs with Partner Countries' HIV/AIDS Strategies and Promote Partner Country Ownership. GAO-10-836. Washington, D.C.: September 20, 2010.

President's Emergency Plan for AIDS Relief: Partner Selection and Oversight Follow Accepted Practices but Would Benefit from Enhanced Planning and Accountability. GAO-09-666. Washington, D.C.: July 15, 2009.

Global HIV/AIDS: A More Country-Based Approach Could Improve Allocation of PEPFAR Funding. GAO-08-480. Washington, D.C.: April 2, 2008.

Global Health: Global Fund to Fight AIDS, TB and Malaria Has Improved Its Documentation of Funding Decisions but Needs Standardized Oversight Expectations and Assessments. GAO-07-627. Washington, D.C.: May 7, 2007.

Global Health: Spending Requirement Presents Challenges for Allocating Prevention Funding under the President's Emergency Plan for AIDS Relief. GAO-06-395. Washington, D.C.: April 4, 2006.

Global Health: The Global Fund to Fight AIDS, TB and Malaria Is Responding to Challenges but Needs Better Information and Documentation for Performance-Based Funding. GAO-05-639. Washington, D.C.: June 10, 2005.

Global HIV/AIDS Epidemic: Selection of Antiretroviral Medications Provided under U.S. Emergency Plan Is Limited. GAO-05-133. Washington, D.C.: January 11, 2005.

Global Health: U.S. AIDS Coordinator Addressing Some Key Challenges to Expanding Treatment, but Others Remain. GAO-04-784. Washington, D.C.: June 12, 2004.

Global Health: Global Fund to Fight AIDS, TB and Malaria Has Advanced in Key Areas, but Difficult Challenges Remain. GAO-03-601. Washington, D.C.: May 7, 2003.

GAO's Mission	The Government Accountability Office, the audit, evaluation, and investigative arm of Congress, exists to support Congress in meeting its constitutional responsibilities and to help improve the performance and accountability of the federal government for the American people. GAO examines the use of public funds; evaluates federal programs and policies; and provides analyses, recommendations, and other assistance to help Congress make informed oversight, policy, and funding decisions. GAO's commitment to good government is reflected in its core values of accountability, integrity, and reliability.
Obtaining Copies of GAO Reports and Testimony	The fastest and easiest way to obtain copies of GAO documents at no cost is through GAO's website (www.gao.gov). Each weekday afternoon, GAO posts on its website newly released reports, testimony, and correspondence. To have GAO e-mail you a list of newly posted products, go to www.gao.gov and select "E-mail Updates."
Order by Phone	The price of each GAO publication reflects GAO's actual cost of production and distribution and depends on the number of pages in the publication and whether the publication is printed in color or black and white. Pricing and ordering information is posted on GAO's website, http://www.gao.gov/ordering.htm. Place orders by calling (202) 512-6000, toll free (866) 801-7077, or TDD (202) 512-2537. Orders may be paid for using American Express, Discover Card, MasterCard, Visa, check, or money order. Call for additional information.
Connect with GAO	Connect with GAO on Facebook, Flickr, Twitter, and YouTube. Subscribe to our RSS Feeds or E-mail Updates. Listen to our Podcasts. Visit GAO on the web at www.gao.gov.
To Report Fraud, Waste, and Abuse in Federal Programs	Contact: Website: www.gao.gov/fraudnet/fraudnet.htm E-mail: fraudnet@gao.gov Automated answering system: (800) 424-5454 or (202) 512-7470
Congressional Relations	Katherine Siggerud, Managing Director, siggerudk@gao.gov, (202) 512-4400, U.S. Government Accountability Office, 441 G Street NW, Room 7125, Washington, DC 20548
Public Affairs	Chuck Young, Managing Director, youngc1@gao.gov, (202) 512-4800 U.S. Government Accountability Office, 441 G Street NW, Room 7149 Washington, DC 20548

Please Print on Recycled Paper.

www.ingramcontent.com/pod-product-compliance
Lightning Source LLC
Chambersburg PA
CBHW080904290526
45795CB00007BA/2399